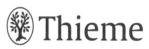

Pediatric Ophthalmology Surgery and Procedures

Tricks of the Trade

Sylvia H. Yoo, MD
Assistant Professor of Ophthalmology
Pediatric Ophthalmology and Strabismus
New England Eye Center
Tufts Medical Center
Boston, Massachusetts, USA

142 illustrations

Thieme
New York • Stuttgart • Delhi • Rio de Janeiro

Library of Congress Cataloging-in-Publication Data is available with the publisher.

Important note: Medicine is an ever-changing science undergoing continual development. Research and clinical experience are continually expanding our knowledge, in particular our knowledge of proper treatment and drug therapy. Insofar as this book mentions any dosage or application, readers may rest assured that the authors, editors, and publishers have made every effort to ensure that such references are in accordance with **the state of knowledge at the time of production of the book**.

Nevertheless, this does not involve, imply, or express any guarantee or responsibility on the part of the publishers in respect to any dosage instructions and forms of applications stated in the book. **Every user is requested to examine carefully** the manufacturers' leaflets accompanying each drug and to check, if necessary, in consultation with a physician or specialist, whether the dosage schedules mentioned therein or the contraindications stated by the manufacturers differ from the statements made in the present book. Such examination is particularly important with drugs that are either rarely used or have been newly released on the market. Every dosage schedule or every form of application used is entirely at the user's own risk and responsibility. The authors and publishers request every user to report to the publishers any discrepancies or inaccuracies noticed. If errors in this work are found after publication, errata will be posted at www.thieme.com on the product description page.

Some of the product names, patents, and registered designs referred to in this book are in fact registered trademarks or proprietary names even though specific reference to this fact is not always made in the text. Therefore, the appearance of a name without designation as proprietary is not to be construed as a representation by the publisher that it is in the public domain.

© 2021. Thieme. All rights reserved.

Thieme Medical Publishers, Inc.
333 Seventh Avenue, New York, NY 10001 USA
+1 800 782 3488, customerservice@thieme.com

Cover design: Thieme Publishing Group
Typesetting by TNQ Technologies, India

Printed in USA by King Printing Company, Inc.   5 4 3 2 1

ISBN 978-1-68420-228-7

Also available as an e-book:
eISBN 978-1-68420-229-4

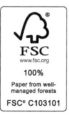

FSC
www.fsc.org
100%
Paper from well-managed forests
FSC® C103101

Contents

10. Botulinum Toxin Injection for Strabismus 71
Sylvia H. Yoo

Section II: Orbital Procedures

11. Nasolacrimal Duct Probing, Intubation, and Balloon Dilation 77
Catherine S. Choi and Maanasa Indaram

Section VI: Examination Under Anesthesia

Preface

The contributors and I took on this project with Thieme to put together a practical and structured guide for pediatric eye surgeries commonly performed by pediatric ophthalmologists. The book will be useful for medical trainees, including medical students, residents, and fellows, to become familiar with the principles and steps of the surgeries before encountering them in the operating room. It will also be useful for surgeons to review the tips and pearls given by the contributors, especially when planning a less-frequently performed procedure. Each section is written by an author with extensive training and experience in the field and provides advanced tips for the procedures described. Alternatives to select procedures are also discussed. Because pediatric ophthalmologists are essentially comprehensive ophthalmologists for infants, children, and teenagers, the book includes procedures within the ophthalmic surgical subspecialties that may be performed by pediatric ophthalmologists.

The first section on strabismus is comprised of ten chapters. The first chapter includes the major goals and principles of all strabismus surgeries, and the subsequent chapters address surgical anatomy for strabismus and the specific surgical steps for various strabismus procedures. Strabismus surgery techniques that are primarily performed in adult patients are not included in this section. The remaining sections cover orbital, anterior segment, glaucoma, and retina procedures. The final chapter on the examination under anesthesia provides organized guidance on preparing for the examination, so that all required equipment and testing are arranged and ready by the time the child is placed under anesthesia. Thieme's *Tricks of the Trade* series, covering a wide range of subspecialties, is subdivided into sections that address goals, advantages, expectations, key principles, indications, contraindications, preoperative preparation, operative technique, tips and pearls, what to avoid, complications, and postoperative care. Pertinent figures and tables are provided to enhance the understanding of the step-by-step descriptions of the procedures.

To continued learning —
Sylvia H. Yoo, MD
Winter 2020, in the midst of the COVID-19 pandemic

Acknowledgments

We are grateful to have had inspiring mentors during our training and early careers who motivated us to take on challenging cases and surgeries and also to pursue our careers in ophthalmology. We also acknowledge our patients, as well as our residents, who open our eyes to novel ways of thinking about and approaching eye diseases every day.

We especially thank:
Steven Archer
Kim Cooper
Monte Del Monte
David Guyton, whose techniques for strabismus surgery, including all of his ingenious intricacies, I am enormously grateful to have learned during my training

David Hunter
Shelley Klein, orthoptist extraordinaire
Hee-Jung Park
Stacy Pineles
Michael Repka
Mitchell Strominger
Deborah VanderVeen
Federico Velez
David Walton

We also thank Ramy Rashad, Allison Resnick, Theodore Lui, and Brandon Pleman for their help with collecting many of the intraoperative photographs included in the book.

Sylvia H. Yoo, MD

Contributors

Alison B. Callahan, MD
Assistant Professor of Ophthalmology
Oculofacial Plastic Surgery
New England Eye Center
Tufts Medical Center
Boston, Massachusetts, USA

Catherine S. Choi, MD
Assistant Professor of Ophthalmology
Pediatric Ophthalmology and Strabismus
New England Eye Center
Tufts Medical Center
Boston, Massachusetts, USA

Shilpa J. Desai, MD
Assistant Professor of Ophthalmology
Vitreoretinal Disease and Surgery
New England Eye Center
Tufts Medical Center
Boston, Massachusetts, USA

Maanasa Indaram, MD
Assistant Professor of Ophthalmology
Pediatric Ophthalmology and Strabismus
University of California-San Francisco
San Francisco, California, USA

Michelle C. Liang, MD
Assistant Professor of Ophthalmology
Vitreoretinal Disease and Surgery
New England Eye Center
Tufts Medical Center
Boston, Massachusetts, USA

Helen H. Yeung, MD
Attending Staff Physician
Department of Ophthalmology
Massachusetts Eye and Ear Infirmary
Boston, Massachusetts, USA

Sylvia H. Yoo, MD
Assistant Professor of Ophthalmology
Pediatric Ophthalmology and Strabismus
New England Eye Center
Tufts Medical Center
Boston, Massachusetts, USA

Section I

Strabismus Surgery

1 Preparation for Strabismus Surgery

Sylvia H. Yoo

Summary

The presence of strabismus precludes normal visual development in infancy and early childhood, resulting in poor fusion and, in many cases, amblyopia. Quality of life can also be affected, especially as the child grows older. Refractive correction and amblyopia treatment may improve strabismus in some children, so that strabismus surgery is not needed. In other cases, strabismus may persist, worsen, or develop, despite nonsurgical treatments or due to other underlying etiologies. Children with constant or poorly controlled deviations larger than 10 to 12 prism diopters can benefit from strabismus surgery not only to improve the ocular alignment but also to improve the chances of developing or maintaining fusion. Diplopia rarely occurs in young children due to suppression of the deviating eye, while older children may report diplopia if the strabismus is worsening or is of new-onset.

The preoperative evaluation of a patient with strabismus includes a complete sensorimotor examination to determine a diagnosis with a clear plan for treatment, which may or may not include strabismus surgery. If strabismus surgery is planned, the goals and risks of surgery are discussed with the patient's family and with the patient, if capable of giving assent. In the operating room, patient and surgeon positioning, coordination with the anesthesiologist, and availability of the proper equipment, instruments, and sutures are key factors to ensure as smooth a surgical experience as possible.

The chapters of this section cover the types of strabismus surgery that may be considered in the pediatric population. Overarching information on the goals, advantages, expectations, indications, contraindications, complications, and postoperative care for strabismus surgery is included in this chapter. Information specific to the type of strabismus surgery described is included in each respective chapter.

Keywords: sensorimotor examination, quality of life, anesthesia, positioning, surgical prep, instruments

1.1 Goals

- The ideal outcome of strabismus surgery is orthophoria in all gaze positions while wearing the appropriate refractive correction to allow development and maintenance of fusion and normal stereoacuity; however, this may not be a realistic surgical outcome in all patients.
- Therefore, the goal of strabismus surgery is an improvement of the ocular alignment, in some cases with a small residual deviation within monofixation range that can allow for development of gross fusion and stable long-term alignment.
- In some cases, improvement of an anomalous head position is the primary goal of strabismus surgery.
- Resolution of diplopia, if present.

1.2 Advantages

- Strabismus surgery is a well-studied treatment for children who have persistent strabismus despite nonsurgical treatments, or for whom nonsurgical treatments are unlikely to improve the eye alignment.
- Observation can be considered an alternative to strabismus surgery but it does not allow for development or maintenance of fusion in early visual development.
- Unlike adults with diplopia due to strabismus, prism glasses are seldom prescribed for strabismus in young children due to suppression and absence of diplopia in most cases.
- In most cases, strabismus surgery can result in stable, long-term improvement of alignment with a favorable risk-to-benefit ratio.
- Compared to botulinum toxin injection, strabismus surgery is less dependent on the presence of or potential for fusion to achieve a good postoperative outcome; if strabismus recurs after botulinum toxin treatment, strabismus surgery is often considered as the next step. Botulinum toxin injection has its own advantages as an alternative to strabismus surgery and is addressed in Chapter 10.

1.3 Expectations

- Safe and effective procedure.
- Improvement of ocular alignment.
- Improvement of stereoacuity in some patients.
- Uncomplicated healing of the operative muscles and conjunctival wounds.

1.4 Key Principles

- The extraocular muscles can be weakened, tightened, and transposed using various methods to improve ocular alignment.
- Proper surgical technique minimizes bleeding and scarring to allow for uncomplicated wound healing and less complex reoperations, should they be needed.

1.5 Indications

The indications for strabismus surgery in the pediatric age range are:

- Abnormal visual development due to strabismus, for which strabismus surgery is performed to increase the chance of normal visual development in early childhood by establishing or re-establishing binocular fusion and treating amblyopia[1] in some patients.
- Strabismus affecting quality of life due to its effects on interpersonal relationships, communication, and self-esteem.[2]
- An anomalous head position due to ocular torticollis from Duane or other dysinnervation syndrome, nystagmus with a null point that is not in primary gaze,[3] or cranial nerve paresis.
- Binocular diplopia.

1.6 Contraindications

- Most patients can safely undergo multiple strabismus surgeries, keeping in mind the following risks:
  - Risk of anterior segment ischemia if two or more rectus muscles in one eye have been previously disinserted. Signs of anterior segment ischemia include conjunctival injection, corneal edema, iritis, iris atrophy, corectopia, posterior synechiae, and cataract formation.
  - Persistent significant misalignment despite multiple strabismus surgeries may indicate that the risks of additional surgery, though low, may actually outweigh the potential benefits, and other treatment options, including observation, may need to be offered. Orbital imaging may be useful in such cases. For example, restriction due to extensive scarring or dysinnervation syndromes with anomalous extraocular muscles may limit the improvement that can be achieved with additional strabismus surgery.
- High general anesthesia risk, in which case the decision for surgery is a collaborative decision with the patient's pediatrician, the anesthesiology team, and the patient's family. If anesthesia is required for another procedure, an effort should be made to combine procedures to avoid multiple episodes of general anesthesia.
- If the patient family's postoperative expectations do not seem realistic, additional discussion is needed and a second opinion may be offered.

1.7 Preoperative Preparation

A detailed history of the presenting strabismus is obtained, including onset (infantile or acquired), frequency of deviation, fixation preference, and any significant anomalous head position. Older children and teenagers may complain of diplopia. A full past medical history, including the patient's birth and developmental history, as well as family history of amblyopia and strabismus are obtained. The family may recall a relative with a "lazy eye," which should be further elaborated.

A complete ophthalmologic examination is performed in the evaluation of strabismus with attention to the sensorimotor examination. The examination begins with testing of stereoacuity and fusion before any dissociation from occlusion during visual acuity and cover testing. Strabismus measurements and visual acuity testing are then performed. If visual acuity testing determines the presence of amblyopia, treatment with refractive correction and/or occlusion therapy may be indicated. In some cases, strabismus surgery that improves eye alignment may also aid in the treatment of amblyopia.[1]

The overall appearance of the patient's eye alignment is observed first. Strabismus measurements are then performed with simultaneous prism cover testing to determine the manifest strabismus, followed by alternate prism cover testing in all gaze positions at distance, and in primary gaze and/or slight downgaze at near.[4] Patterns such as V- or A-patterns may be noted during the measurements and may be correlated to oblique muscle overaction during evaluation of versions. Measurements in right and left head tilt are also performed if a cyclovertical strabismus is present. Additional latent strabismus may be revealed by prism adaptation testing or prolonged cover testing to maximally dissociate the patient. In poorly cooperative patients and young infants, cover testing in only primary gaze at near or corneal light reflex testing with or without prisms may be used to estimate the deviation. Conversely, older children with vertical strabismus and complaints of torsional diplopia, may undergo double Maddox rod testing or Lancaster red-green testing to evaluate torsion. In addition, in older children with possible anomalous retinal correspondence who are at risk of developing early postoperative diplopia, which typically resolves, a loose prism can be used during preoperative testing to demonstrate the type of diplopia they may experience in the early postoperative period to help set expectations.

Versions and ductions are then evaluated with attention to overaction or underaction of the horizontal and cyclovertical extraocular muscles and in more extreme gaze positions than may be examined during prism testing. Forced duction testing can be performed at the time of surgery under anesthesia to confirm suspected restriction as a cause of strabismus and, in some cases, for final surgical planning. During the office examination, the patient's head position is also observed. An anomalous head position may be due to an incomitant strabismus resulting from Duane syndrome or other dysinnervation syndrome, cranial nerve paresis or palsy, nystagmus with a null point not in primary gaze, and even due to refractive error in some children. The examination then proceeds with dilation of the pupils and cycloplegia to measure the cycloplegic refraction and to perform a fundoscopic examination. If a significant refractive error is found, refractive correction may be warranted before proceeding with strabismus surgery.

Examination findings which indicate a possible systemic or neurologic cause of strabismus should be further investigated with imaging and possibly blood work in coordination with the patient's pediatrician.

1.8 Surgical Planning

The planning for strabismus surgery and the surgery itself are embodiments of the art of medicine. While uncomplicated cases may have one straightforward approach for treatment, many cases have more than one option for a favorable outcome. The surgery that is performed depends on the preoperative and intraoperative examination findings, as well as the surgeon's experience.

The subsequent chapters of this section will address in detail the various ways to weaken, tighten, or transpose the extraocular muscles. In some patients with prior ocular surgery or injury, surgery on the extraocular muscles may not always be

required; rather, dissection and release of adhesions and scarring around the extraocular muscles may be sufficient to resolve restriction causing the strabismus.

1.9 Perioperative Tips and Pearls

1.9.1 Anesthesia

General anesthesia is required for strabismus surgery, including brief procedures, in pediatric patients. Communication should occur with the anesthesiology team regarding concerns about underlying medical problems including acute upper respiratory infections, a family history of malignant hyperthermia, and preferred preoperative fasting guidelines.[5] Child life specialists are also a part of the multimodal approach to prepare the pediatric patient for surgery. Families may ask about concerns for neurotoxicity from anesthesia exposure in young children. At this time, they may be reassured that, while the effects of anesthesia on a child's development remain unclear, the initial concern was based on animal studies using very high doses of anesthetic agents, and recent human studies are reassuring.[5] In addition, a short duration of anesthesia, which is sufficient for most strabismus surgeries, appears safer than long-duration or repetitive exposures.

A laryngeal mask airway (LMA) may be used in most patients. Some patients with chronic diseases and syndromes may be at increased risk of anesthesia related complications, including difficult airways, hemodynamic instability due congenital heart disease, and metabolic abnormalities, and endotracheal intubation with paralysis may be safer for these patients,[5] as well as for young infants. The distal end of the LMA or endotracheal tube should lie as flat as possible on the patient's chin and chest, so that it does not tent the surgical drape and remains directed away from the surgical field, decreasing the risk of dislodgement. Propofol anesthesia has the advantage of causing less postoperative nausea, but strabismus surgery in itself increases the risk of nausea. Postoperative pain and nausea may be mitigated by the use of perioperative medications, including ketorolac, dexamethasone, ondansetron, and acetaminophen, in coordination with the anesthesiologist. During surgery, the surgeon should notify the anesthesiologist when traction is to be placed on an extraocular muscle, especially a rectus muscle, to be prepared for potential changes in the heart rate secondary to the oculocardiac reflex. Communication regarding signs that additional anesthesia is needed, based on observations of the patient's Bell's reflex or unexpected movement, or when the second eye surgery is about to begin, can also ensure efficiency in the operating room and patient safety.

1.9.2 Positioning

An eye gurney with a head rest is used for optimal positioning of the surgeon, assistant, and patient. The patient's neck should be slightly hyperextended for better access to the eye, with the top of the head positioned at the top of the head rest.[6] The gurney is rotated during the surgery so that the anesthesiologist is monitoring the patient from the side, rather than at the head of the patient. Once the patient is under anesthesia, the gross eye alignment can be briefly assessed by opening both eyelids before prepping and draping the surgical field.

For the horizontal rectus muscles, the surgeon is seated to the side of the patient's head with the assistant sitting across from the surgeon. The surgeon has the best view and access to the operative muscle by sitting opposite to the side of the horizontal rectus muscle insertion; for example, for left lateral rectus surgery, the surgeon is positioned on the right side of the patient's head.[7] Some surgeons may be comfortable operating on either side of the head for horizontal rectus muscle surgery. For superiorly inserted muscles, the surgeon sits on the side of the operative eye, facing superiorly. For inferiorly inserted muscles, the surgeon sits at the head of the bed. For the cyclovertical muscles, the assistant sits approximately 90 degrees away from the surgeon, toward the side of the operative eye. The assistant's hands and arms should remain out of the surgeon's working field, for example, by draping the forearm near the top of the patient's head and under the surgeon's hands (▶ Fig. 1.1). The surgical instrument tray is positioned over the patient's body or at the head of the bed, depending on the surgeon's preference.

1.9.3 Prepping and Draping

The surgical site(s) is marked prior to arrival to the operating room. The brows, eyelids, nasal bridge, and upper cheeks are prepped using 5% povidone-iodine solution, which may be lightly dabbed after application and then allowed to dry for disinfection and for the drapes to adhere properly. Attention is

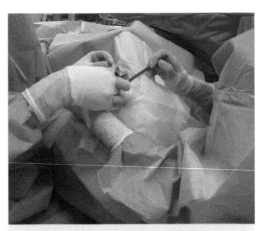

Fig. 1.1 The assistant's hands and arms should remain out of the surgeon's working field by draping the forearm near the top of the patient's head and under the surgeon's hands and arms. In this figure, the surgeon is seated on the left, and the assistant is on the right.

given to the eyelid margins and eyelashes, where meibum, debris, and bacteria can accumulate. Several drops of povidone-iodine should also be instilled into the operative eye(s) as well. In patients who are truly allergic to iodine, dilute hypochlorous acid solution 0.01 to 0.02% may be used. Chlorhexidine solution should not be used in or around the eye. One drop of phenylephrine 2.5% can then be instilled for vasoconstriction. Various methods of draping can be used to ensure maintenance of a sterile field and adequate exposure of the surgical field. One method of draping is as follows. A sterile towel covers the airway to avoid inadvertently dislodging the tube when the drapes are removed. A small surgical drape is used to cover the forehead and top of the head, and a large drape to cover the lower face and body. Over these drapes, a nonfenestrated clear plastic drape with a rectangular area of adhesive is placed over the eyes while using the distal ends of sterile cotton-tip applicators to open the eyelids so that the lashes are covered by the adhesive portion of the drape (▶ Fig. 1.2a). Alternative methods of draping depend on the surgeon's preference and availability of drapes at the hospital or surgical center. For example, ▶ Fig. 1.2b shows the use of a fenestrated clear drape over sterile towels and a large U-drape. The nonfenestrated drape is opened with blunt-tipped scissors by using the tips of the closed blades to create an opening near the medial canthus (▶ Fig. 1.3) and then extending the opening as a slit temporally to create room for an appropriately-sized speculum, with care

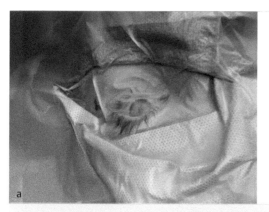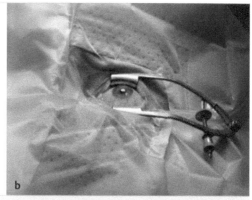

Fig. 1.2 (a) One method of draping the patient for strabismus surgery: A nonfenestrated clear plastic drape with an area of adhesive covers the drapes over the patient's head and body, with cotton-tip applicators used to open the eyelids and position the lashes out of the surgical field. **(b)** Alternatively, a fenestrated drape can be used over sterile towels and a U-drape. A closed eyelid speculum is then used to position the lashes out of the surgical field.

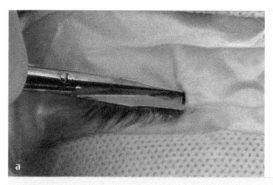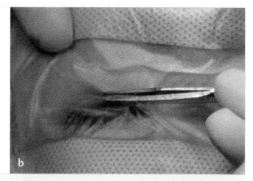

Fig. 1.3 (a) The drape is opened with blunt-tipped scissors near the medial canthus and **(b)** extended temporally.

to avoid cutting lashes or skin. If bilateral surgery is planned, the drape can be opened for both eyes to perform forced ductions bilaterally for comparison. This comparison is especially important for the oblique muscles. The fellow eye can then be covered and kept moist by carefully reapproximating the drape closed with a sterile sticker label, so that the lashes remain tucked under the clear drape. Once the first eye procedure is complete, the drape over the first eye is lifted to allow the eye to close, and attention is directed to the second eye for surgery by removing the sticker label and placing an eyelid speculum.

1.9.4 Instruments and Supplies

Suggested sutures, medications, and instruments are listed in ▶ Table 1.1. with brief descriptions of their uses during strabismus surgery. A suggested set-up for the surgical instrument tray is shown in ▶ Fig. 1.4. Surgical loupes with 1.5–2.5 × magnification, keeping in mind the field of view and working distance for head and neck positioning, are used for strabismus surgery. Overhead surgical lights should be adjusted to illuminate the operative eye and muscles during the surgery. A headlight is helpful during cyclovertical muscle surgery to better direct light posteriorly and can also be used during postoperative adjustments.

1.10 What to Avoid

- Excessive manipulation of tissue which can lead to greater bleeding and scar formation.
- Injury to the cornea during surgery.
- Suboptimal location of the conjunctival fornix incision:
  - May affect access to the operative muscle(s).

Table 1.1 Suggested sutures and instruments with brief descriptions of their uses during strabismus surgery

6–0 polyglactin suture, double-armed on spatulated needles	Absorbable suture for reinsertion of operative muscles
6–0 polyester suture, double-armed on spatulated needles	• Nonabsorbable suture for very large rectus muscle recessions and for inferior rectus muscle recessions which otherwise may not adhere to the globe during healing • Used as a traction suture for the adjustable suture technique • Used as a suture spacer for superior oblique weakening surgery and for superior oblique tuck procedures • Used for posterior fixation
6–0 or 7–0 fast-absorbing or chromic gut suture	If sutured closure of conjunctival incision is needed; 8–0 polyglactin suture may also be used
Stevens tenotomy hooks	Two small hooks for initial hooking of extraocular muscles and for exposure of the operative field
Jameson muscle hooks	Two large hooks with a bulbed tip to securely hook the extraocular muscles and for rectus muscle resections
Guyton muscle hook	To securely hook the extraocular muscle and to maintain a small conjunctival incision
Wright grooved hook, left and right	Decreases the risk of scleral perforation during imbrication of extraocular muscles, especially for tight muscles; once the suture is in place, the Wright hook may be replaced by a Guyton hook or Jameson hook for more room during disinsertion
Gass hook	To safely tag muscles with a 4–0 silk suture, which can also be used for traction
Manson double hook	For exposure of the operative field
Toothed forceps	Three 0.3- or 0.5-mm Castroviejo forceps for forced duction testing and to grasp the conjunctiva and sclera; the tips of the forceps may be inspected at the start of the case to ensure that the teeth are in good condition for securely holding tissue
Locking toothed forceps	Two 0.5-mm Castroviejo locking forceps may be used to lessen the need for a surgical assistant by being able to simultaneously hold the eye in position and provide adequate exposure of the operative field
Bipolar jeweler forceps or handheld cautery pen	For cautery of vessels at the scleral insertion site once a muscle is disinserted; to cauterize a muscle before resection and during inferior oblique myectomy. The setting for bipolar cautery may be machine-dependent, but a level of 4 may be used as a starting point. Note that handheld cautery is very hot while the tip is red and may be best used just after the redness diminishes
Non-toothed forceps for conjunctiva	For delicate handling of the conjunctiva
Hartman straight mosquito clamp	For hemostasis before a rectus muscle is resected and to clamp the inferior oblique before disinsertion and myectomy
Bulldog serrefine clamps	Can be used to hold sutures away from the surgical field
Fine locking curved needle drivers	Three needle drivers for holding needles and suture
Fine nonlocking curved needle driver	Some surgeons prefer to use a nonlocking needle driver for partial-thickness scleral passes, during which the swaged end of the needle, though not sharp, may perforate the globe if a locking needle driver is inadvertently still locked during reloading of the needle as it is passed
Blunt Westcott scissors	For blunt and sharp dissection of conjunctiva and connective tissue; for rectus muscle disinsertion, some surgeons prefer right and left Aebli corneal section scissors
Stevens tenotomy scissors	Blunt-tipped scissors to create a slit in the clear drape
Eyelid speculum	A wire or closed blade speculum of appropriate size for the patient
Small Desmarres or Conway retractor	For posterior exposure, such as during superior rectus, inferior rectus, and oblique muscle surgery
Malleable ribbon retractor	Helpful for far posterior exposure, such as during placement of posterior fixation sutures
Castroviejo calipers	To measure the amount of recession or resection

Table 1.1 *(Continued)* Suggested sutures and instruments with brief descriptions of their uses during strabismus surgery

Straight metal ruler	May be used to confirm that the calipers are properly calibrated
Scott curved ruler	To measure very large recessions and for posterior fixation
Iris spatula	For rectus muscle plications
Bishop tendon tucker	For superior oblique tuck procedures
Balanced salt solution with irrigation cannula	To maintain lubrication of the cornea; sterile lubricating ointment or a moist corneal sponge may also be used

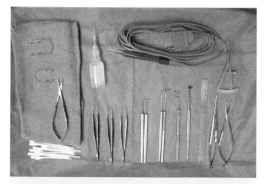

Fig. 1.4 Suggested set-up for the surgical instrument tray for strabismus surgery.

- Incisions should be kept anterior to the extraconal fat pad.
- May result in inadequate coverage of the muscle suture at the conclusion of surgery, affecting postoperative healing.
- Tearing of the conjunctival incision, which is less of a concern in the pediatric age range than in older adult patients.
- Splitting the operative muscle with a muscle hook.
- Imbricating the muscle too close or too far from where it will be disinserted or resected
- Repeated partial-thickness scleral passes, which increases the risk of scleral perforation and may decrease the integrity of the new insertion site.

1.11 Complications

Undercorrection and overcorrection, sometimes requiring additional strabismus surgery, are the primary risks to underscore during the preoperative discussion, with the understanding that this can occur soon after surgery or, in some cases, years later. Additional risks[8] to discuss include:
- Diplopia in the early postoperative period, which usually resolves in primary gaze earlier than in side gazes.

- Suture allergy, epithelial inclusion cyst, or granuloma, which can be treated with a topical corticosteroid in most cases or may require excision of the suture or granuloma if persistent.
- Excessive scar formation or fat adherence syndrome.
- Infection:
  - Preseptal or orbital cellulitis requiring systemic antibiotic treatment.
  - Endophthalmitis is a rare complication of strabismus surgery and requires a high index of suspicion and early evaluation and treatment, in collaboration with a vitreoretinal specialist.
- Slipped or lost muscle, requiring additional surgery to recover the muscle.
- Anterior segment ischemia, especially if more than two to three rectus muscles are disinserted in one eye.
- Scleral perforation due to a deep needle pass during reinsertion of the muscle.
  - If suspected during surgery, a dilated fundus examination is performed to evaluate for evidence of a retinal break; if present, cryotherapy is performed, and the patient is likely to have more postoperative pain than typical for strabismus surgery.
  - Retinal detachment can also occur and must be urgently referred to a vitreoretinal specialist for evaluation and treatment.
  - Endophthalmitis can also be a complication of scleral perforation.
- Surgical errors, including wrong eye and wrong muscle procedures, as well as recession versus resection error.
- Risks of general anesthesia including nausea and vomiting; more serious risks of anesthesia are rare in healthy patients.

1.12 Postoperative Care and Expectations

- For most patients, strabismus surgery is an outpatient procedure, not requiring overnight hospital admission.

- Redness of the eyes improves within 1 to 2 weeks but may take several weeks to completely resolve.
- Crusting and mild discharge, as well as pink or blood-tinged tears in the early postoperative period, can be cleaned with a soft washcloth.
- Activity restrictions:
  - Children may return to normal activities including daycare or school within 1 week after surgery. Rubbing the eyes may be inevitable, but most children can be discouraged from rubbing the eyes and are unlikely to rub so vigorously to cause damage, as forceful rubbing is likely to cause more discomfort.
  - Teenagers are recommended to avoid regular activities including school for approximately 1 week, and avoid rigorous exercise or heavy lifting of more than 10 pounds for 1 week.
  - Bathing or showering is safe, keeping water out of the eyes as ordinarily would be done; swimming in a pool or other body of water should be avoided for 1 week after surgery.
- The need to continue glasses and/or amblyopia treatment postoperatively should be reviewed with the family.
- No eye pads or shields are needed after strabismus surgery.
- A topical combination antibiotic and corticosteroid eyedrop or ointment is used for 1 to 2 weeks after strabismus surgery.
- Patients with an underlying immune disorder may be prescribed a systemic antibiotic preoperatively and also given an intravenous antibiotic intraoperatively.
- Over-the-counter pain medications such as acetaminophen and ibuprofen may be used and should provide adequate pain control. If pain is more severe, the surgeon should be notified. Resections and reoperations may cause more discomfort than recessions and surgery on previously unoperated muscles. Postoperative opioids are rarely needed after discharge, but codeine and hydrocodone should be avoided, as they are prodrugs with variable metabolism. A limited supply of oxycodone is more suitable if needed.[5]
- The first postoperative visit may occur 1 to 2 weeks after surgery and then in 2 to 3 months to evaluate the final alignment.
- More frequent or earlier visits may be required if there are unexpected events or findings. Return precautions should be provided on a written handout for the patient's family to review if any concerns should arise, including a sudden change in alignment with poor eye movement, severe or worsening eye pain with associated redness of the eyes or swelling of the eyelids, or changes in vision.

References

[1] Lam GC, Repka MX, Guyton DL. Timing of amblyopia therapy relative to strabismus surgery. Ophthalmology. 1993; 100 (12):1751–1756

[2] Nelson BA, Gunton KB, Lasker JN, Nelson LB, Drohan LA. The psychosocial aspects of strabismus in teenagers and adults and the impact of surgical correction. J AAPOS. 2008; 12(1): 72–76.e1

[3] Mitchell PR, Wheeler MB, Parks MM. Kestenbaum surgical procedure for torticollis secondary to congenital nystagmus. J Pediatr Ophthalmol Strabismus. 1987; 24(2):87–93

[4] Mehta A. Chief complaint, history and physical examination. In: Rosenbaum AL, Santiago AP, eds. Clinical Strabismus Management: Principles and Surgical Techniques. Philadelphia, PA: Saunders Company; 1999:3–21

[5] Waldschmidt B, Gordon N. Anesthesia for pediatric ophthalmologic surgery. J AAPOS. 2019; 23(3):127–131

[6] Wright KW. Color Atlas of strabismus surgery: strategies and techniques, 3rd ed. New York, NY: Springer; 2007

[7] Del Monte MA, Archer SM. Atlas of pediatric ophthalmology and strabismus surgery. New York, NY: Churchill Livingstone; 1993

[8] Wan MJ, Hunter DG. Complications of strabismus surgery: incidence and risk factors. Semin Ophthalmol. 2014; 29(5–6):421–428

2 Surgical Anatomy for Strabismus Surgery

Sylvia H. Yoo

Summary

Understanding the anatomy of the rectus and oblique muscles and their relationships to adjacent structures are essential to approaching strabismus surgery for successful outcomes, particularly in reoperations or congenital anomalies in which the normal anatomy has been altered or is abnormal.

Keywords: rectus muscles, oblique muscles, spiral of Tillaux, Tenon's capsule, anterior ciliary arteries, vortex veins

2.1 Extraocular Rectus and Oblique Muscles

Six extraocular muscles control the motility of each eye: the medial and lateral rectus muscles, the superior and inferior rectus muscles, and the superior and inferior oblique muscles (► Fig. 2.1). The four rectus muscles arise from the annulus of Zinn, a tendinous ring which encloses the optic foramen and a section of the medial superior orbital fissure. All six extraocular muscles insert on the eye, where the associated anterior ciliary arteries may be more easily identified subconjunctivally than the muscles themselves. The insertions of the rectus muscles form the spiral of Tillaux (► Fig. 2.2) according to their distances from the limbus. They are approximately 7 mm apart, and are slightly curved, so that the central insertion is closest to the limbus.[1] Foot plates, which are small attachments of the rectus muscle to the sclera, may be present just posterior to the insertions. While the functions of the horizontal rectus muscles are straightforward as adductors and abductors, the

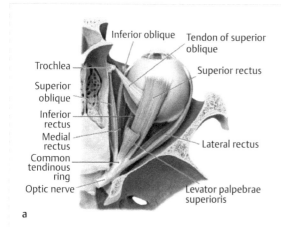

Trochlea
Superior oblique
Inferior rectus
Medial rectus
Common tendinous ring
Optic nerve
Inferior oblique
Tendon of superior oblique
Superior rectus
Lateral rectus
Levator palpebrae superioris

a

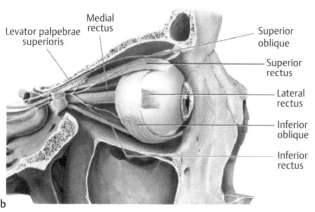

Levator palpebrae superioris
Medial rectus
Superior oblique
Superior rectus
Lateral rectus
Inferior oblique
Inferior rectus

b

Fig. 2.1 The six extraocular muscles, from their origins to their insertions on the eye—(a) superior view and (b) lateral sagittal view. (Reproduced with permission from Schünke M, Schulte E, Schumacher U. Thieme Atlas of Anatomy: Head, Neck and Neuroanatomy, 2nd ed. Stuttgart: Thieme; 2016.)

11

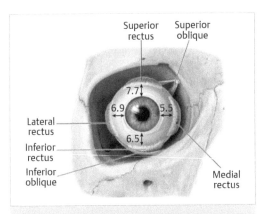

Fig. 2.2 The rectus muscle insertions form the spiral of Tillaux, with the medial rectus closest to the limbus, and the superior rectus furthest from the limbus (right eye pictured, measurements in millimeters). (Reproduced with permission from Schünke M, Schulte E, Schumacher U. Thieme Atlas of Anatomy: Head, Neck and Neuroanatomy, 2nd ed. Stuttgart: Thieme; 2016.)

functions of the cyclovertical muscles are more complex due to their paths of action, which are diagonal to the visual axis when the eye is in primary gaze. Understanding the relationships of the functions of the cyclovertical muscles is useful for surgical planning in patients with vertical and torsional strabismus. See ▶ Table 2.1 and ▶ Table 2.2 for detailed anatomic and functional features of each muscle.

2.2 Conjunctiva and Sclera

The landmarks of the conjunctiva are used when creating conjunctival incisions for strabismus surgery. Medially located incisions should avoid the plica semilunaris to avoid excessive scarring, bleeding, and pain.[2] Identification of the plica may be affected by conjunctival follicles commonly seen in children. The caruncle is less likely to be injured due to its far nasal location, but its position may shift with large medial rectus resections. In the inferior fornix, extraconal fat can be identified as a raised yellow area, starting at approximately 10 mm posterior to the limbus and should not be disrupted.

The sclera is thinnest at 0.3 mm just posterior to the rectus muscle insertions. This area of thin sclera can be visualized intraoperatively and in some patients with prior rectus muscle recessions as a gray area posterior to the original insertion.

2.3 Subconjunctival Fascia

The Tenon's capsule covers the entire sclera, fusing with the optic nerve sheath posteriorly and with the conjunctiva and sclera 1 to 3 mm from the limbus, so that the extraocular muscles pass through the capsule approximately 10 mm posterior to the limbus to reach their insertions on the sclera.[3] Thus, a rectus muscle transposition is limited by the location of the Tenon's capsule opening because the posterior path of the muscle does not significantly change. The Tenon's capsule separates extraconal fat from the sclera posteriorly and from the sclera and extraocular muscles anteriorly.

Each rectus muscle is surrounded by a fascial capsule, which is dissected intraoperatively for exposure of the tendon and muscle, and secure suture placement. The fibroelastic muscle pulley system also surrounds the rectus muscles and stabilizes the paths and positions of the muscles, possibly acting as the mechanical origins of the muscles.[4] The anterior pulley system, made up of the intermuscular septum and the check ligaments between the muscle sheath and the anterior Tenon's capsule, can be identified during dissection of the extraocular muscles.

2.4 Vascular Structures

In most people, seven anterior ciliary arteries provide the blood supply to the anterior segment of each eye. Two vessels are associated with each of the rectus muscles except the lateral rectus, which usually has one associated anterior ciliary artery. Anteriorly, these vessels are visible on the surface of the muscle within the fascial capsule, usually located near each edge of the muscle, with the lateral rectus vessel near the inferior edge. The vessels usually branch into a cluster of vessels and emerge at the poles of the muscles onto the sclera, forming an episcleral plexus, which may bleed easily when dissecting to bare sclera at the insertion of the muscle. Once disrupted, the anterior ciliary arteries rarely re-canalize but with time, collateral circulation may develop, although the risk of anterior segment ischemia remains.

The four vortex veins emerge from the sclera posteriorly, approximately 16 mm posterior to the limbus and are susceptible to injury during strabismus surgery on the cyclovertical muscles, especially during posterior dissection due to their locations near the vertical rectus and oblique muscles.

Table 2.1 Extraocular muscle anatomy: origin, insertion, size, arc of contact

Muscle	Origin	Insertion	Size	Arc of contact (in mm)
Medial rectus	Annulus of Zinn, medial and inferior to the optic foramen	5.5 mm from the limbus	Muscle is 40.8 mm long Tendon is 3.7–4.5 mm long, 10.3 mm wide	6–7
Inferior rectus	Annulus of Zinn, inferior to the optic foramen	6.5 mm from the limbus	Muscle is 40 mm long Tendon is 5.5–7 mm long, 9.8 mm wide	6.5–7
Lateral rectus	Annulus of Zinn, spanning the superior orbital fissure	6.9 mm from the limbus	Muscle is 40.6 mm long Tendon is 7–8 mm long, 9.2 mm wide	10–12
Superior rectus	Annulus of Zinn, superior and lateral to the optic foramen, inferior to the origin of the levator palpebrae superioris	7.7 mm from the limbus	Muscle is 41.8 mm long Tendon is 5.8 mm long, 10.6 mm wide	6.5
Superior oblique	Superomedial to the optic foramen, near the origin of the levator palpebrae superioris Functional origin is the trochlea located on the orbital rim at the anterior superomedial orbit on the frontal bone	Muscle becomes tendon just before the trochlea, then continues laterally and posteriorly under the superior rectus, passing through the Tenon's capsule 2 mm nasal and 5 mm posterior to the nasal insertion of the superior rectus muscle and inserting on the posterior super-otemporal quadrant of the eye behind the equator, 12–13 mm posterior to the limbus with a fan-like insertion which is parallel to the lateral margin of the superior rectus muscle and with anterior fibers oriented circum-ferentially	Muscle is 32–40 mm long Tendon is 20–26 mm long, 10–18 mm wide with a cord-like segment as it passes from the trochlea under the nasal aspect of the superior rectus and then fans out into a wide insertion	8–12
Inferior oblique	Maxillary bone, infero-lateral to the lacrimal sac fossa, just posterior to the orbital rim, may partially arise from the lacrimal sac fascia	Posterior inferotemporal quadrant in the area of the macula 10% have two muscle bellies	Muscle is 37 mm long and 9.6 mm wide at its insertion Tendon is minimally present	15

Sources: Data from Glasgow BJ. Anatomy of the Human Eye. Mission for Vision. http://www.images.missionforvisionusa.org/anatomy/2005/10/eye-anatomy-human.html (published 2005; accessed November 1, 2019) and Lueder GT, Archer SM, Hered RW, et al. Basic and Clinical Science Course: Pediatric Ophthalmology and Strabismus. San Francisco, CA: American Academy of Ophthalmology; 2014.

Table 2.2 Extraocular muscle anatomy: blood supply, innervation, relationship to adjacent structures, actions

Muscle	Blood supply	Innervation	Relationship to adjacent structures	Actions
Medial rectus	Inferior/medial muscular branch of ophthalmic artery, giving rise to two anterior ciliary arteries	Inferior division of third cranial nerve (oculomotor nerve) on its lateral surface at the junction of its medial and posterior thirds	No fascial attachments to oblique muscles Passes through the Tenon's capsule 12 mm posterior to its insertion	Adduction
Inferior rectus	Inferior/medial muscular branch of ophthalmic artery and infraorbital artery, giving rise to two anterior ciliary vessels	Inferior division of third cranial nerve (oculomotor nerve) on its upper surface at the junction of the middle and posterior thirds	Attached to lower eyelid by fascial expansion of its sheath, 15–18 mm posterior to its insertion Muscle sheaths of the inferior oblique and inferior rectus muscles combine to form Lockwood's ligament from which the capsulopalpebral fascia, the major retractor of the lower eyelid, extends and travels parallel to the inferior rectus before inserting at the inferior tarsus Inferonasal and inferotemporal vortex veins are near the nasal and temporal edges of the inferior rectus posteriorly	Primary depression (sole depressor in abduction) Secondary extorsion Tertiary adduction Also depresses the lower eyelid
Lateral rectus	Lacrimal artery and/or superior/lateral muscular branch of the ophthalmic artery, giving rise to one anterior ciliary artery (may vary)	Sixth cranial nerve (abducens nerve) on its medial surface just posterior to the middle of the muscle	Connection with inferior oblique at the inferior oblique insertion	Abduction
Superior rectus	Superior/lateral muscular branch of the ophthalmic artery, giving rise to two anterior ciliary arteries	Superior division of the third cranial nerve (oculomotor nerve) under the muscle at the junction of the middle and posterior thirds	Fascial connections with the levator palpebrae superioris Connection to underlying superior oblique tendon Superonasal and superotemporal vortex veins are near the nasal and temporal edges of the superior rectus posteriorly	Primary elevation (sole elevator in abduction) Secondary intorsion Tertiary adduction Also helps elevate the upper eyelid
Superior oblique	Superior/lateral muscular branch of the ophthalmic artery	Fourth cranial nerve (trochlear nerve) at its superolateral aspect of the posterior third of the muscle	Trochlea-tendon complex: Trochlea is U-shaped and fibro-cartilaginous, tendon and its fibrovascular sheath move through the trochlea like a telescope While variable, the anterior aspect of the insertion is approximately 3–5 mm posterior to the temporal pole of the superior rectus muscle insertion, while the posterior aspect of the	Primary intorsion (primarily anterior one-third fibers) Secondary depression (posterior two-thirds fibers, sole depressor in adduction)

Table 2.2 (*Continued*) Extraocular muscle anatomy: blood supply, innervation, relationship to adjacent structures, actions

Muscle	Blood supply	Innervation	Relationship to adjacent structures	Actions
			insertion is 13–14 mm posterior to the superior rectus muscle insertion, so that the superior oblique insertion is approximately 11 mm wide. Superotemporal vortex vein is near the posterior aspect of the superior oblique tendon insertion	Tertiary abduction (posterior two-thirds fibers)
Inferior oblique	Inferior/medial muscular branch of the ophthalmic artery and infraorbital artery	Inferior division of the third cranial nerve (oculomotor nerve) at the posterior and upper aspect, approximately 15 mm nasal to the insertion, within a neurovascular bundle	In contact with the periosteum of the orbital floor near its origin, then separated from the floor laterally by orbital fat and covered by the lateral rectus and Tenon's capsule Muscle sheaths of the inferior oblique and inferior rectus muscles combine to form Lockwood's ligament, which may act as the effective insertion of the muscle in inferior oblique weakening procedures. With inferior oblique anteriorization, the neurovascular bundle may act as the effective origin Inferotemporal vortex vein loops along the posterior border of the inferior oblique	Primary extorsion Secondary elevation (sole elevator in adduction) Tertiary abduction

Sources: Data from Glasgow BJ. Anatomy of the Human Eye. Mission for Vision. http://www.images.missionforvisionusa.org/anatomy/2005/10/eye-anatomy-human.html (published 2005; accessed November 1, 2019) and Lueder GT, Archer SM, Hered RW, et al. Basic and Clinical Science Course: Pediatric Ophthalmology and Strabismus. San Francisco, CA: American Academy of Ophthalmology; 2014.

References

[1] Glasgow BJ. Anatomy of the human eye: mission for vision. http://www.images.missionforvisionusa.org/anatomy/2005/10/eye-anatomy-human.html. Published 2005. Accessed November 1, 2019

[2] Wright KW. Color Atlas of strabismus surgery: strategies and techniques, 3rd ed. New York, NY: Springer; 2007

[3] Del Monte MA, Archer SM. Atlas of pediatric ophthalmology and strabismus surgery. New York, NY: Churchill Livingstone; 1993

[4] Demer JL. Mechanics of the orbita. Dev Ophthalmol. 2007; 40:132–157

3 Conjunctival Incisions for Strabismus Surgery

Sylvia H. Yoo

Summary

Fornix and limbal conjunctival incisions have superseded the Swan incision for accessing the extraocular muscles during strabismus surgery.

Fornix incisions will be the primary technique for strabismus surgery discussed throughout this section. The limbal incision will be also be described in this chapter.

Keywords: fornix incision, limbal incision, Tenon's capsule

3.1 Goals

- Minimize postoperative discomfort and scarring of the conjunctiva following strabismus surgery with a well-positioned and well-approximated conjunctival incision.

3.2 Advantages

Limbal conjunctival incisions allow greater exposure of the rectus muscle and surrounding structures, especially for reoperations and complex strabismus, and is more easily performed without a trained surgical assistant. However, a well-placed fornix incision has several advantages:

- The incision and conjunctival scar are hidden by the upper or lower eyelid.
- The incision does not require sutured closure in most cases, reducing surgical time and patient discomfort, except in the following scenarios:
  - The incision tears or extends to the limbus.
  - The patient has an underlying immune disorder.
  - The incision does not adequately cover the operative muscle and muscle suture.
  - Surgeon's preference.
- If sutured closure of the fornix incision is required, the sutures are located away from the limbus for less discomfort and foreign body sensation, which can occur after closure of a limbal incision.
- Avoid scarring of the conjunctiva and Tenon's capsule to the sclera anterior to the rectus muscle insertion to improve cosmesis and decrease the difficulty of reoperations if needed.
- One incision allows access to multiple extraocular muscles:

- An inferonasal fornix incision can access the medial rectus and the inferior rectus muscles.
- An inferotemporal fornix incision can access the lateral rectus and inferior rectus muscles, as well as the inferior oblique muscle.
- Inferior quadrant incisions are typically used for horizontal rectus muscle surgery.
- A superonasal incision can access the medial rectus and superior rectus muscles, as well as the nasal aspect of the superior oblique tendon.
- A superotemporal incision can access the medial rectus and superior rectus muscles, as well as the temporal aspect and insertion of the superior oblique tendon.
- Fornix incisions should be used for oblique muscle surgery.
- Radially oriented fornix incisions heal with little visible conjunctival scarring, but if greater exposure is required or if there is concern that the conjunctiva may tear easily, a circumferential fornix incision can be used, although the conjunctival scar may be slightly more visible by the surgeon after the incision heals.
- With the use of locking toothed forceps, strabismus surgery with a fornix incision can be performed without a trained surgical assistant, as the locking forceps can be used to position the eye and provide exposure of the surgical field simultaneously.
- The perilimbal conjunctiva may contribute to the anterior segment blood supply, so that a fornix incision preserves these anastamoses, possibly decreasing the risk of anterior segment ischemia.[1]

3.3 Expectations

- Coverage of the operative extraocular muscle and its suture by the conjunctiva at the conclusion of surgery.
- Little to no discomfort postoperatively, apart from reoperations with significant scarring.

3.4 Key Principles

- Fornix incisions are created in the quadrant of the globe that provides access to the operative extraocular muscle(s).
- Limbal incisions require sutured closure, which may cause more discomfort due to the presence

of suture near the limbus, and can increase the risk of corneal dellen formation.

3.5 Indications

- Fornix incisions can be used for most strabismus surgeries in the pediatric population.
- If conjunctival scarring overlying a rectus muscle is causing restriction, a conjunctival recession may be indicated, which requires a limbal incision.

3.6 Contraindications

Patients with a history of multiple strabismus surgeries resulting in extensive scarring, or other prior ocular surgeries with placement of extraocular implants such as scleral buckles or glaucoma tube shunts, may necessitate limbal incisions for greater exposure of the operative muscle(s) and surrounding structures.

3.7 Preoperative Preparation

The decision for the type and location of the incision is made based on the planned operative muscle(s) and the patient's ocular surgical history.

3.8 Operative Technique

3.8.1 Fornix Incision

The fornix incision is actually located on the bulbar conjunctiva between rectus muscles and becomes hidden in the fornix. Minimal scar formation occurs between the conjunctiva and Tenon's capsule to the sclera, making reoperations less difficult if needed.

- An eyelid speculum is placed. The eye is grasped with a 0.3-mm toothed forceps at the limbus, in the intermuscular quadrant where the incision is to be made, and then rotated to expose the quadrant.
- The exposed quadrant of conjunctiva is inspected to ensure that it is not overlying a rectus muscle. Approximately 6 to 8 mm from the limbus, the conjunctiva is grasped and tented with two pairs of toothed forceps which are positioned circumferentially for creation of a radial incision (▶ Fig. 3.1a). For a circumferential incision parallel to the eyelid margin, one or two pairs of forceps may be used to tent the conjunctiva.
- Blunt Westcott scissors are positioned between the pairs of forceps on the conjunctiva with the blunt tips flushed against the globe and then snipped to create a conjunctival incision (▶ Fig. 3.1b). If the first snip of the Westcott scissors does not reveal bare sclera, the forceps are used again to grasp the underlying Tenon's capsule to create an incision, preferably at a 90-degree angle from the conjunctival incision.
- The blades of the blunt Westcott scissors are closed and used to bluntly dissect the intermuscular space to bare sclera, orienting the curve of the blades with the curvature of the globe and keeping the blades open while withdrawing the scissors (▶ Fig. 3.2).

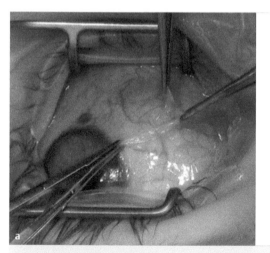
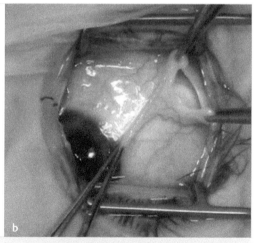

Fig. 3.1 (a) The inferotemporal conjunctiva is tented with forceps for the blades of Westcott scissors to be oriented radially across the tented conjunctiva. **(b)** A radial fornix incision in the inferotemporal quadrant.

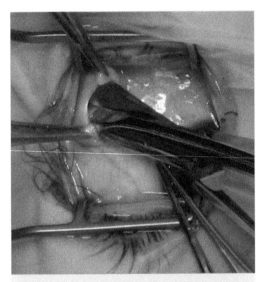

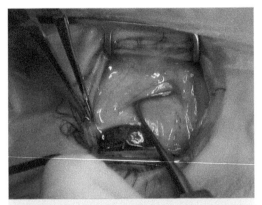

Fig. 3.3 The fornix incision is reapproximated by grasping the eye with forceps and massaging the incision closed with a small hook.

Fig. 3.2 Westcott scissors are used to bluntly dissect the intermuscular space to bare sclera, keeping curve of the blades parallel to the curvature of the sclera.

- Once the planned strabismus surgery is completed, the fornix incision can be reapproximated in most cases without sutured closure by grasping the eye at 6 o'clock with toothed forceps for an inferior incision and massaging the incision closed with the heel of a Stevens hook (▶ Fig. 3.3).

3.8.2 Limbal Incision

- An eyelid speculum is placed. The eye is grasped with a 0.3-mm toothed forceps at the limbus, anterior to the operative muscle insertion, and the eye is rotated away from the operative muscle.
- A radial conjunctival incision is made with blunt Westcott scissors in one of the quadrants adjacent to the operative rectus muscle and extended to the limbus.
- A peritomy is then created 1 to 2 mm from the limbus in the quadrant of the operative rectus muscle.
- A second radial relaxing incision can be made on the opposite quadrant of the rectus muscle if additional exposure is needed (▶ Fig. 3.4).
- Blunt Westcott scissors are used to bluntly dissect Tenon's capsule to bare sclera around the rectus muscle, avoiding trauma to the muscle itself.
- Once the planned strabismus surgery is completed, the limbal incision is closed with 8–0 or 9–0 polyglactin suture at the limbal corner(s) of the incision, aiming to bury the knots as much as

possible. The relaxing incisions may be sutured with interrupted sutures if there is a significant gap in the wound.
- Minimally invasive strabismus surgery (MISS) uses multiple small conjunctival incisions for horizontal rectus muscle surgery, requires a surgical microscope, and has a steep learning curve. The incisions for MISS are made where the surgical steps will be performed, away from the limbus and perpendicular to the insertion, with the size of the incision dependent on the planned amount of recession or resection. The incisions can be converted to a limbal incision intraoperatively if greater exposure is needed.[2]

3.9 Tips and Pearls

- When grasping the globe with toothed forceps, orient the forceps perpendicular to the surface of the globe for the teeth to securely grasp the conjunctiva and episcleral tissue.
- The location of a fornix incision should not be too anterior, so that it is hidden by the eyelid and not too far posterior, especially for inferonasal and inferotemporal incisions, as anterior orbital fat can be inadvertently exposed.
- If sutured closure of a fornix incision is required, the incision is reapproximated with forceps, and one to three interrupted sutures are usually needed to close the incision, with the goal of burying the knot and tails of the sutures by first passing the needle inside the incision (▶ Fig. 3.5). The author closes fornix incisions, if needed, with 6–0 or 7–0 fast-absorbing or chromic gut suture, which may result in less inflammation

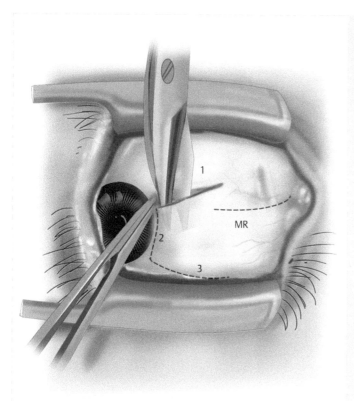

Fig. 3.4 For a limbal incision, a peritomy is made approximately 1 to 2 mm from the limbus with radial relaxing incisions. A nasal incision is pictured for medial rectus (MR) surgery.

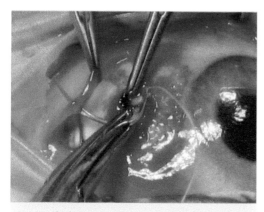

Fig. 3.5 If a fornix incision requires sutured closure, the knots are buried by first passing the needle inside the incision.

and irritation postoperatively compared to polyglactin suture.[3]

- Exposed Tenon's capsule can be judiciously trimmed at the conclusion of surgery if it does not remain tucked under the conjunctival incision and hidden by the eyelid.

- When using a limbal incision, a fine-tipped surgical marker can be used to create two reference marks at the corners of the limbal incision, which may facilitate wound closure.
- When closing a limbal incision, the suture is placed through the corner of the conjunctival flap and then passed through conjunctiva and episclera in the perilimbal area for secure closure.

3.10 What to Avoid

- When a nasal fornix incision is made, ensure that the plica semilunaris and the caruncle are not involved in creation of the conjunctival incision to avoid excessive bleeding and scarring. Temporal conjunctival incisions that extend to the lateral canthus can result in symblepharon formation.
- The Swan incision, made directly over and parallel to the rectus muscle insertion, has been superseded by the incisions described above due to a greater risk of bleeding and inadvertent disinsertion of the muscle, as well as scarring between the conjunctiva and the insertion and underlying muscle.[4]

3.11 Complications

- Exposed Tenon's capsule resolves with continued healing in most cases but can be trimmed in the office for cooperative patients if desired.
- Tenon cyst formation resolves in many cases with a topical steroid and observation, but some cases require surgical excision.
- With limbal incisions or if there is significant chemosis or redundant conjunctiva adjacent to the limbus, especially following a large resection of a rectus muscle, there is risk of corneal dellen formation, which can be treated with aggressive lubrication and typically resolves with continued healing of the conjunctiva.

3.12 Postoperative Care

- If sutured closure of the conjunctival incision is needed, a combination antibiotic and steroid ointment, rather than an eye drop, may be used to ameliorate discomfort or foreign body sensation that may occur.

References

[1] Fishman PH, Repka MX, Green WR, D'Anna SA, Guyton DL. A primate model of anterior segment ischemia after strabismus surgery: the role of the conjunctival circulation. Ophthalmology. 1990; 97(4):456–461

[2] Mojon DS. Review: minimally invasive strabismus surgery. Eye (Lond). 2015; 29(2):225–233

[3] Sridhar J, Kasi S, Paul J, et al. A prospective, randomized trial comparing plain gut to polyglactin 910 (Vicryl) sutures for sclerotomy closure after 23-gauge pars plana vitrectomy. Retina. 2018; 38(6):1216–1219

[4] Wright KW. Color atlas of strabismus surgery: strategies and techniques, 3rd ed. New York, NY: Springer; 2007

4 Rectus Muscle Surgery

Sylvia H. Yoo

Summary

Rectus muscle recessions and resections are the most common strabismus surgeries performed in the pediatric age range, specifically horizontal rectus muscle surgery for esotropia and exotropia. Unilateral or bilateral surgery may be performed, depending on the preoperative evaluation and indications for the procedure. Considerations when performing vertical rectus muscle surgery are also discussed in this chapter. The adjustable suture technique, transpositions, partial tendon procedures, and reoperations are addressed in subsequent chapters.

Keywords: medial rectus, lateral rectus, superior rectus, inferior rectus, recession, hangback recession, resection, plication, esotropia, exotropia, pattern strabismus, hypertropia, Duane syndrome, anomalous head position, nystagmus

4.1 Goals

In addition to the goals of strabismus surgery stated in Chapter 1.1 Goals, the goals of rectus muscle surgery include the following:
- For intermittent exotropia, a small distance overcorrection of 8 to 10 prism diopters in the early postoperative period may improve the probability of long-term improved alignment, although the reported outcomes are variable and likely depend on the patient's sensory status.[1]
- Improvement of eye alignment in primary gaze and/or improvement of an anomalous head position in patients with incomitant strabismus due to Duane syndrome, other dysinnervation syndrome, or cranial nerve palsies.
- With the Anderson-Kestenbaum procedure,[2] improvement of an anomalous head turn in patients with nystagmus and a null point not in primary gaze.
- With superior rectus recessions, improvement of manifest dissociated vertical deviations in patients without inferior oblique overaction or tightness of the inferior oblique muscles on forced duction testing.

4.2 Advantages

- Refractive correction and amblyopia treatment may improve control of certain types of strabismus, including accommodative esotropia and intermittent exotropia. For those patients with constant or poorly controlled misalignment, strabismus surgery is offered as a treatment to improve the alignment. Strabismus surgery on the rectus muscles is likely to be more effective than botulinum toxin injection in patients with poor potential for fusion.
- For rectus muscle recessions, the muscle can be reinserted with direct scleral passes at the new insertion site or at the original insertion using a hangback technique:
  - The hangback technique is useful for very large recessions, especially of the superior rectus muscle because far posterior scleral passes could interfere with the superior oblique tendon.[3]
  - The hangback technique may also be preferred by inexperienced strabismus surgeons, including trainees, as the insertion is more easily accessible, possibly reducing the risk of scleral perforation.
  - However, the hangback technique may result in a larger recession than intended due to central sag and may increase the risk of stretch scar formation, which can lead to recurrent strabismus.[4]
- An alternative to a small resection is rectus muscle plication, which appears to preserve the anterior ciliary circulation, as the muscle is not disinserted.[5]

4.3 Expectations

- Diplopia, typically transient, may occur in the early postoperative period, usually due to anomalous retinal correspondence and sometimes due to early overcorrection and/or surgically induced incomitance.

4.4 Key Principles

- A rectus muscle can be weakened by recessing the muscle and tightened by resecting or plicating

the muscle to improve ocular alignment in patients with horizontal and vertical deviations.
- Resections are tightening procedures, not strengthening procedures. Large resections can even result in restriction of ocular motility, which may be desired in some cases.
- For bilateral procedures in children, bilateral recessions are typically performed before resections, depending on the deviation at distance and near, as well as versions and ductions. Unilateral procedures, such as recess-resect procedures, are indicated in some cases.

4.5 Indications

- Various etiologies of strabismus may be treated with rectus muscle surgery, including:
  - Comitant esodeviations and exodeviations, including partially accommodative esotropia, nonaccommodative esotropia, infantile esotropia or exotropia, and intermittent exotropia.
  - Sensory esodeviations and exodeviations for which unilateral surgery is recommended.
  - Dissociated vertical deviations.
  - Congenital dysinnervation syndromes including Duane syndrome and monocular elevation deficiency.
  - Oculomotor nerve (3rd cranial nerve) palsies.
  - Abducens nerve (6th cranial nerve) palsies.
  - Restrictive strabismus.
- Patients with nystagmus and a null point not in primary gaze, resulting in an anomalous head turn.

4.6 Contraindications

In patients who have a prior history of strabismus surgery on two to three rectus muscles in one eye, the increased risk of anterior segment ischemia is considered when planning the timing of and approach for subsequent strabismus surgery.

4.7 Preoperative Preparation

A complete sensorimotor examination is performed as discussed in Chapter 1.7 Preoperative Preparation. Surgical planning takes into consideration the amount of deviation, presence of amblyopia in determining the laterality of surgery, the presence of pattern strabismus, as well as forced duction testing under anesthesia before the start of surgery, especially if restriction is suspected.

- Horizontal deviations with V- or A-patterns without significant oblique muscle overaction can be addressed with vertical displacement of pairs of horizontal rectus muscles during reinsertion of the muscle. This is less commonly performed in unilateral recess-resect procedures, as patients with normal fusion may develop torsional diplopia, although it can be considered in those with limited fusion.[6] The mnemonic M-A-L-E is commonly used to recall the direction of displacement. For example, for a V-pattern, if the bilateral Medial rectus muscles are the operative muscles, they are infraplaced (toward the Apex of the "V"). If the bilateral Lateral rectus muscles are the operative muscles, they are supraplaced (toward the Empty space of the "V"). Understanding the rationale for this effect is advantageous for recalling how the muscles should be displaced for pattern horizontal strabismus (▶ Fig. 4.1).[3] For example, when the lateral rectus muscles are recessed and supraplaced for a V-pattern exotropia, the muscles are effectively further recessed when the eye is in upgaze to treat the larger exodeviation in upgaze. Without changing the planned amount of recession or resection for the horizontal deviation in primary gaze, half-tendon-width to full-tendon-width displacements, depending on the difference in the deviation in upgaze and downgaze, may be used, or the amount of displacement may be measured in millimeters.
- A small vertical deviation, such as one caused by a partial oculomotor nerve (3rd cranial nerve) paresis, can also be addressed with vertical displacements of the horizontal rectus muscles. For example, supraplacement of horizontal rectus muscles can effectively pull a hypotropic eye upward. Approximately 1 mm of displacement corrects 1 prism diopter of vertical deviation for up to 10 prism diopters.
- In Duane syndrome, rectus muscle resections in the involved eye are usually avoided due to the risk of worsening restriction and globe retraction. In patients with severe globe retraction with or without an upshoot or downshoot, recessions of both the medial and lateral rectus muscles may be considered. In esotropic Duane syndrome, large recessions of the medial rectus muscles are usually needed for significant improvement of the deviation and head turn. Forced ductions prior to the start of surgery should be performed.

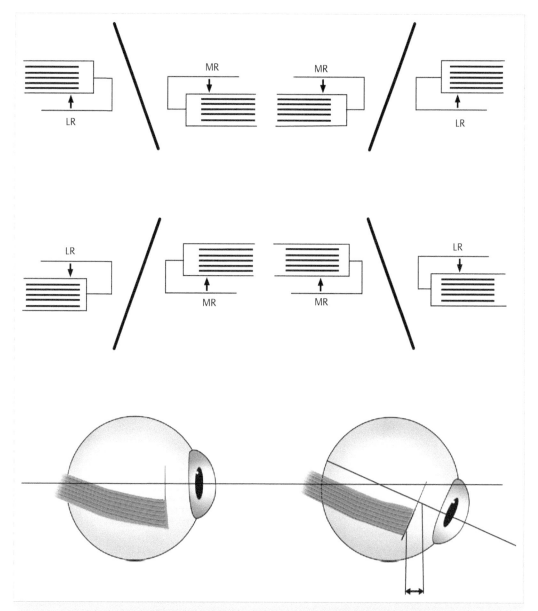

Fig. 4.1 Vertical displacement of the horizontal rectus muscles is used to treat V-pattern and A-pattern horizontal strabismus. LR, lateral rectus; MR, medial rectus.

- Dissociated vertical deviation (DVD) is a bilateral but often asymmetric form of strabismus. Thus, bilateral surgery is recommended in most cases, except in patients who are unable to alternate fixation due to a very strong fixation preference, usually due to significantly decreased visual acuity in one eye. Otherwise, unilateral surgery for an asymmetric DVD will unveil the DVD in the unoperated eye, requiring additional surgery.

4.8 Operative Technique

Guidelines for the amounts of surgery to perform for the horizontal rectus muscles based on preoperative measurements are given in ▶ Table 4.1.[7] Several tables are available for horizontal rectus muscle surgery which vary more for larger deviations and are less reliable for reoperations, restrictive and paretic strabismus, and dysinnervation syndromes.

Table 4.1 Guidelines for the amounts of horizontal rectus surgery to perform based on preoperative measurements

Deviation (prism diopters)	Esotropia			Exotropia		
	Bilateral medial rectus recession (millimeters)	Medial rectus recession (millimeters)	Lateral rectus resection (millimeters)	Bilateral lateral rectus recession (millimeters)	Lateral rectus recession (millimeters)	Medial rectus resection (millimeters)
15	3.0	3.0	4.0	4.0	4.0	3.0
20	3.5	3.5	5.0	5.0	5.0	4.0
25	4.0	4.0	6.0	6.0	6.0	5.0
30	4.5	4.5	7.0	7.0	7.0	6.0
35	5.0	5.0	8.0	7.5	7.5	6.5
40	5.5	5.5	9.0	8.0	8.0	7.0
50	6.0	6.0	10.0	9.0	9.0	7.5
60	6.25	6.25	11.0	10.0	10.0	8.0

Source: Data from Guyton DL. Strabismus: History, principles, surgical anatomy, surgical options and indications. In: Gottsch JD, Stark WJ, Goldberg MF, eds. Ophthalmic Surgery, 5th ed. London: Arnold; 1999:64–72.
Note: Horizontal deviations greater than 50 to 60 prism diopters are best treated with three or four muscle surgery extrapolated from the table to decrease the risk of limiting ductions with very large recessions and resections.

Table 4.2 Amounts of superior rectus surgery for dissociated vertical deviations

Deviation (prism diopters)	Bilateral superior rectus recession (mm)
Less than 10	6.0
10–15	8.0
15–20	9.0
Greater than 20	10.0

Source: Data adapted from Rosenbaum AL, Santiago AP, eds. Clinical Strabismus Management: Principles and Surgical Techniques. Philadelphia, PA: Saunders Company; 1999.

Table 4.3 Horizontal rectus muscle surgery to perform for a right or left head turn in patients with a right or left head turn due to nystagmus with a null point not in primary gaze

Degrees of head turn	20 degrees	20–45 degrees	45 degrees
Right head turn			
Right medial rectus recession	6.0 mm	6.5 mm	7.0 mm
Right lateral rectus resection	9.5 mm	10.5 mm	11.25 mm
Left medial rectus resection	7.25 mm	7.75 mm	8.5 mm
Left lateral rectus recession	8.5 mm	9.0 mm	9.75 mm
Left head turn			
Right medial rectus resection	7.5 mm	7.75 mm	8.5 mm
Right lateral rectus recession	8.5 mm	9.0 mm	9.75 mm
Left medial rectus recession	6.0 mm	6.5 mm	7.0 mm
Left lateral rectus resection	9.5 mm	10.5 mm	11.25 mm

Source: Data from Cestari DM, Hunter DG, eds. Learning Strabismus Surgery: A Case-Based Approach. Philadelphia, PA: Lippincott Williams & Wilkins; 2013.

For the vertical rectus muscles, 1 mm of recession or resection corrects for approximately 3 prism diopters of deviation, usually with a recommended maximum of 5 mm of surgery. However, larger recessions of the superior rectus muscles are typically required to effectively treat dissociated vertical deviations (▶ Table 4.2).[8] ▶ Table 4.3[9] displays the amounts of surgery to perform for patients with a large right or left head turn due to nystagmus with a null point that is not in primary gaze, also known as the Anderson-Kestenbaum procedure. This procedure is typically performed in school-age children or older. When deliberating which muscles to recess and resect for this procedure, the adducted eye can be considered "esotropic" and the abducted eye "exotropic," while allowing the preferred head turn. The large amounts of surgery used, particularly the resections, can result in limitations of postoperative ductions, which is part of the desired effect of this procedure. If strabismus is also present, the surgical numbers are modified. One method for surgical planning for a patient with strabismus and a head turn due to

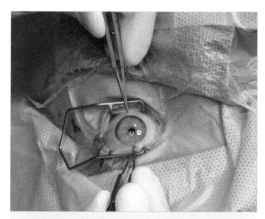

Fig. 4.2 For forced duction testing of the horizontal rectus muscles, the eye is grasped at 12 and 6 o'clock near the limbus, and the eye is gently proptosed.

nystagmus is to place a loose prism over the fixating eye until the head turn resolves. While keeping the first prism in place, the strabismus is then measured with prisms over the nonfixating eye.

4.8.1 Forced Duction Testing

For forced duction testing of the horizontal rectus muscles, two pairs of 0.3- or 0.5-mm toothed forceps are used to grasp the eye at 12 and 6 o'clock near the limbus (▶ Fig. 4.2). The eye is gently proptosed, as retropulsion of the globe places the rectus muscles on slack and can give a false negative result. The eye is adducted and abducted to evaluate for tightness of the medial and lateral rectus muscles. For the vertical rectus muscles, the eye is grasped at 3 and 9 o'clock. If a pattern strabismus is present, exaggerated traction testing of the oblique muscles is also performed, as described in Chapter 6.8.1 Exaggerated Traction Testing.

Following the creation of a fornix incision, as described in Chapter 3.8.1 Fornix Incision, the steps for rectus muscle surgery are described below.

4.8.2 Isolating the Operative Muscle

1. The eye continues to be grasped at the limbus, and the conjunctival incision is held open with forceps. A Stevens hook is used to isolate the operative rectus muscle with the handle nearly perpendicular to the insertion (▶ Fig. 4.3a), keeping in mind the approximate location of the insertion from the limbus. Once the muscle

is securely hooked, the assistant can release the forceps from the limbus, while keeping the conjunctival incision open with forceps.

2. A Jameson hook is then used to sweep along the muscle insertion just posterior to the Stevens hook, which is subsequently removed (▶ Fig. 4.3b). A Guyton hook may subsequently be used to hook the muscle in a similar manner, after which the Jameson hook is removed.

3. The bulb of the Guyton or Jameson hook is swept to nearly reach the limbus subconjunctivally as an early test to confirm that the entire width of the muscle has been isolated. If not, toothed forceps can be used to gently grasp the muscle through the conjunctiva to bring the entire muscle onto the hook.

4. Point the bulb of the Guyton or Jameson hook slightly away from the globe to gather the width of the muscle in the elbow of the hook and use a Stevens hook to drape the overlying conjunctiva over the bulb of the Guyton or Jameson hook. Care should be taken during this part of the procedure to avoid either unhooking the muscle or tearing the conjunctiva. Also ensure that the conjunctiva is not folded over the bulb of the hook before snipping the intermuscular septum in the next step to avoid creation of a buttonhole in the conjunctiva.

5. Blunt Westcott scissors are used to snip the intermuscular septum just under the bulb of the Guyton or Jameson hook until an opening is created (▶ Fig. 4.4a). The assistant should retract the conjunctiva away from the bulb of the Guyton or Jameson hook with a small hook to expose the intermuscular septum. The closed blades of the Westcott scissors, a small hook, or toothed forceps are then used to expose the bulb of the Guyton or Jameson hook through the opening of the intermuscular septum (▶ Fig. 4.4b).

6. A pole test is now performed to confirm that the entire width of the muscle has been isolated. The assistant and the surgeon each place a Stevens hook in the opening of the intermuscular septum with both hooks oriented so that the tips are flushed on the sclera. One hook holds open the incision, and the second hook performs the pole test by sweeping the tip from posterior to the insertion, around the pole of the insertion, to anterior to the insertion (▶ Fig. 4.5). If the hook does not easily slide anteriorly and comes to a stop at the plane of the insertion, the muscle has likely been split. The split portion of the muscle can be hooked with

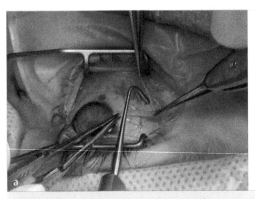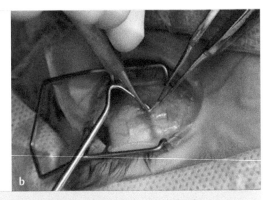

Fig. 4.3 **(a)** A small hook is first used to isolate the operative muscle, **(b)** followed by the Jameson hook.

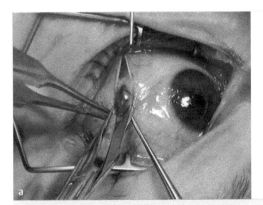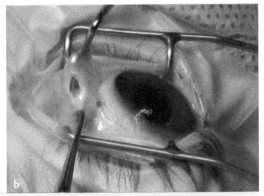

Fig. 4.4 **(a)** The intermuscular septum is incised under the bulb of the Guyton hook, **(b)** then the bulb of the hook can be exposed through the opening of the intermuscular septum.

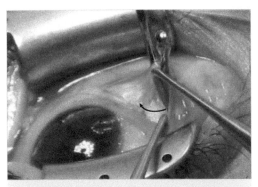

Fig. 4.5 The pole test is performed by the surgeon and the assistant using two small hooks, with one hook holding the incision open, and the tip of the second hook sliding from posterior to the insertion, around the pole of the insertion, to anterior to the insertion (*arrow*).

a small hook and brought onto the Guyton or Jameson hook to re-join the split muscle. Step 5 is repeated, followed by the pole test. The pole test can also be performed on the opposite pole of the muscle in the same manner.

7. The two Stevens hooks are then used by the assistant to tent the overlying conjunctiva to expose the muscle (▶ Fig. 4.6), Tenon's capsule, and check ligaments which are bluntly and sharply dissected using blunt Westcott scissors while taking care not to cut the muscle.

8. One Stevens hook is brought anteriorly to retract the conjunctiva away from the insertion to dissect Tenon's capsule to bare sclera, while holding the muscle taut on the Guyton or Jameson hook to visualize the area anterior to the insertion. The Tenon's capsule can be grasped and tented with forceps, and Westcott scissors used to

bluntly clear the Tenon's capsule from sclera (▶ Fig. 4.7a). Once the Tenon's capsule is separated from sclera, it can be sharply dissected off the muscle and sclera, if needed (▶ Fig. 4.7b).

9. The center of the anterior insertion is dried and marked on sclera (▶ Fig. 4.8), keeping in mind any planned vertical displacement for a pattern strabismus.

4.8.3 Rectus Muscle Recession

1. Once the operative muscle is isolated, a 6–0 double-armed polyglactin suture secures the central one-fourth to one-third width of the rectus muscle near its insertion with a central full-thickness 2–1 throw square knot.

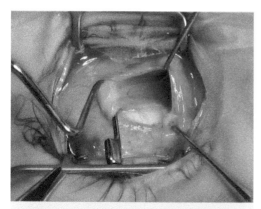

Fig. 4.6 Two small hooks tent the overlying conjunctiva to bluntly dissect Tenon's capsule and the check ligaments away from the muscle using Westcott scissors.

2. Each end of the suture is passed partial thickness with a slight weaving motion through the respective half to one-third of the muscle width to the edge of the muscle (▶ Fig. 4.9), followed by a full-thickness pass including one-fourth to one-third of the muscle width. The suture is then locked by passing the end of the suture with the needle through the loop that is created at the edge of the muscle (▶ Fig. 4.10a) and tightened (▶ Fig. 4.10b).

3. Both ends of the suture are then gathered and held taut between the thumb and forefinger while the same hand holds the Guyton or Jameson hook between the forefinger and the middle finger (▶ Fig. 4.11).

4. Blunt Westcott scissors are used to disinsert the muscle with consecutive small snips flush to the sclera (▶ Fig. 4.12), leaving a small stump that can be grasped securely without cutting the muscle suture. Foot plates posterior to the insertion may be present and are also disinserted. The sutures are then released.

5. The insertion is grasped with toothed forceps and cotton-tip applicators are used to dry the insertion and identify bleeding vessels. Minimal cautery is used to cauterize the vessels, aiming for the vessels at and just anterior to the insertion and avoiding cautery posterior to the insertion where the sclera is thinner. A Stevens hook is used by the assistant to retract the conjunctiva away from the insertion.

6. The rectus muscle can then be reinserted with either direct scleral passes at the new insertion site or at the original insertion using a hangback technique.

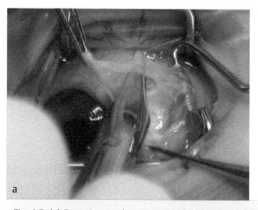

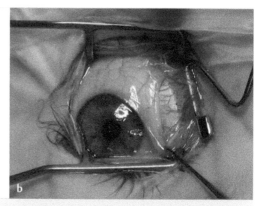

Fig. 4.7 **(a)** Tenon's capsule anterior to the insertion is bluntly dissected with toothed forceps and Westcott scissors, while a small hook retracts the conjunctiva. **(b)** Once the Tenon's capsule is cleared, bare sclera and the anterior ciliary arteries are readily visible.

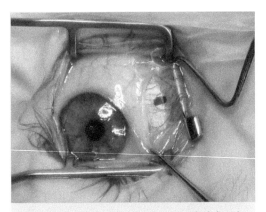

Fig. 4.8 The center of the insertion is marked directly on sclera.

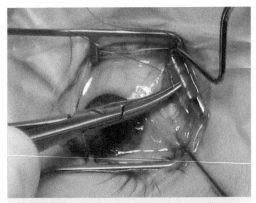

Fig. 4.9 One end of the 6–0 polyglactin suture is passed partial thickness on the rectus muscle, near its insertion, to the edge of the muscle during imbrication for a rectus muscle recession.

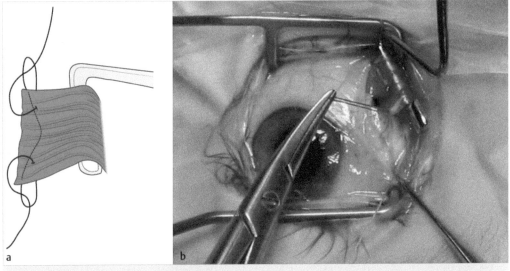

a
b

Fig. 4.10 (a) Following the partial-thickness then full-thickness passes at the edge of the rectus muscle during imbrication, the suture is locked by passing the end of the suture through the loop that is created at the edge of the muscle and **(b)** securely tightened by first pulling taut the segment of suture between the loop and muscle and then pulling the end of the suture.

7. For direct scleral reinsertion, calipers are set at the planned amount of recession in millimeters which may be confirmed with a straight ruler. One tip of the calipers, that is, the side with the knob, is marked with a marking pen:
   a) The insertion is grasped with toothed forceps and the calipers are placed with the un-marked tip at the level of the insertion, either at one pole or with vertical displacement if needed for pattern strabismus or a small vertical deviation. The marked tip is oriented posterior and perpendicular to the insertion. The new insertion site is dried with a cotton-tip applicator and marked (▶ Fig. 4.13). Alternatively, two locking forceps may be used at the insertion and held by the assistant who also retracts the conjunctiva with a Stevens hook for better exposure if needed.
   b) The ends of the suture are held up to identify the poles of the muscles with their respective

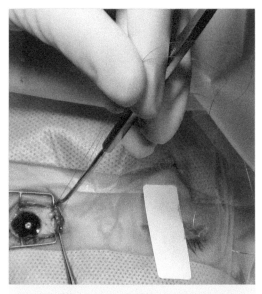

Fig. 4.11 The sutures are held taut with the Guyton or Jameson hook.

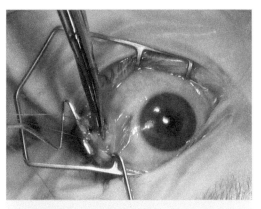

Fig. 4.12 The muscle is disinserted with Westcott scissors with consecutive small snips flush to the sclera, leaving a small stump without cutting the muscle suture.

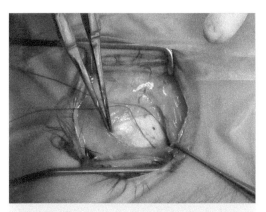

Fig. 4.13 The new insertion site has been marked by marked calipers before direct scleral reinsertion during recession of a rectus muscle.

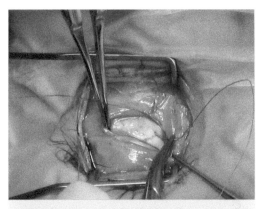

Fig. 4.14 Reinsertion of the muscle with a partial-thickness sclera pass. Note the positioning of the needle, loaded at its center with the sharp end of the needle pointing slightly away from the globe, and the needle visible along its course.

needles, and the end corresponding to the first mark is chosen. The needle is loaded on a needle holder near its center. The insertion is securely grasped with toothed forceps. If needed, a Stevens hook is used by the assistant to provide exposure of the mark, while positioning the hook so that the surgeon's hands are not impeded. The needle is held with its tip oriented tangential to and pointed slightly away from the sclera, then engaged in the sclera at the mark and

carefully advanced partial thickness, ensuring that the needle is visible along the entire scleral tract without being too shallow (▶ Fig. 4.14). The course of the needle may be toward the center of the insertion or may be nearly perpendicular to the insertion.

c) The above two steps are repeated for reinsertion of the opposite pole of the muscle. Again, the assistant retracts the conjunctiva with a Stevens hook if needed.

d) The muscle is pulled up to the new insertion site with both ends of the suture, and a 3–1–1 throw square knot is tied to secure the

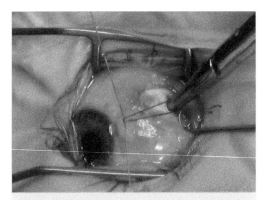

Fig. 4.15 The muscle is tied down at its new insertion with a 3–1-1 throw square knot. To maintain the position of the muscle, the first 3-throw knot can be held with an empty needle holder which is released once the first 1-throw knot is ready to tighten.

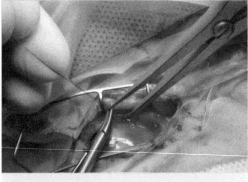

Fig. 4.16 The muscle is pulled up to the original insertion and calipers set at the planned amount of recession are used to measure from the insertion, along the suture toward the needles. Here, an empty needle holder is placed on the suture, just inside the distal tip of the calipers.

muscle. If the muscle is tending to hang back while tying the knot, the first 3-throw tie can be held with an empty needle holder by the assistant and then released once the first 1-throw knot is ready to tighten (▶ Fig. 4.15). Any Tenon's capsule that becomes pulled into in the knot should be released before tightening the knot.

e) The recession distance is confirmed with calipers, and the muscle is evaluated for central sag. If central sag is present, one end of the suture can be passed full thickness through the center of the muscle tendon, passing the needle from the underside of the muscle. The suture is then tied again, pulling the central portion of the muscle in line with the poles.

8. For a hangback recession technique, the needles are reinserted at the original insertion:

a) First, the ends of the suture are held up to identify the poles of the muscles with their respective needles. One end is chosen and the needle loaded on a needle holder near its center. The insertion is securely grasped with toothed forceps. The tip of the needle is then oriented tangential to and pointed slightly away from the sclera. The needle is engaged partial thickness in the sclera at one pole of the original insertion or with vertical displacement if needed for pattern strabismus or a small vertical deviation. The needle may enter the sclera nearly at the base of the small ridge at the original insertion and is then carefully advanced partial thickness

anteriorly, ensuring that the needle is visible along the entire scleral tract without being too shallow. The path of the needle may be directed toward the center of the area anterior to the insertion or perpendicular to the insertion.

b) The above step is repeated for the opposite pole of the muscle. The assistant retracts the conjunctiva with a Stevens hook if needed.

c) The muscle is pulled up to the original insertion with both ends of the suture which are held taut. Calipers set at the planned amount of recession are used to measure from the insertion, along the length of the muscle suture toward the needles. A straight locking needle holder clamps both ends of the suture, just inside the distal tip of the calipers (▶ Fig. 4.16), and a 3–1-1 throw square knot is tied over the needle holder.

d) The needle holder is removed, and the insertion is grasped to rotate the globe away from the muscle so that the muscle hangs back. The needle holder can be used to pull the sutures posteriorly through the scleral tunnels if needed. The recession distance is then confirmed with calipers.

4.8.4 Rectus Muscle Resection

1. Once the operative muscle is isolated on a Guyton hook, a Jameson hook is placed under the muscle posteriorly with the handle in the opposite direction of the Guyton hook (▶ Fig. 4.17). Calipers are set for the planned

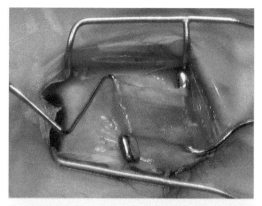

Fig. 4.17 For a rectus muscle resection, a Jameson hook is placed under the muscle posteriorly with the handle in the opposite direction of the Guyton hook.

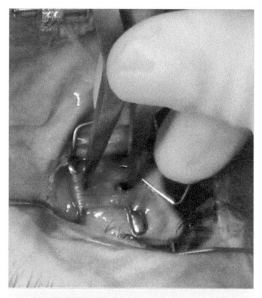

Fig. 4.18 Calipers with one tip marked are used to mark the site of resection on the muscle.

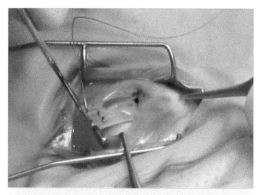

Fig. 4.19 If a rectus muscle plication is planned, the suture is placed to imbricate the muscle posterior to the mark without clamping or cauterizing the muscle at the resection site.

amount of resection and one tip, that is, the side with the knob, is marked. The unmarked tip of the calipers is placed at the insertion and the marked tip is used to mark the site of resection on the muscle with several marks along the width of the muscle (▶ Fig. 4.18).

2. The marked resection site is clamped with a small straight clamp, and then bipolar cautery is placed across the muscle and slowly withdrawn while lightly cauterizing the resection site.

3. A double-armed 6–0 polyglactin suture is used to imbricate the central one-fourth to one-third width of the rectus muscle posterior to the cautery mark with a central full-thickness 2–1 throw square knot. The suture should be placed near the cautery mark to avoid resecting

the muscle more than intended but without the risk of cutting the suture or leaving too narrow an area of tissue, through which the sutures could cheesewire when the muscle is resected.

4. Each end of the suture is passed partial thickness with a slight weaving motion through the respective half to one-third of the muscle width to the edge of the muscle, followed by a full-thickness pass including one-fourth to one-third of the muscle width which is locked by passing the end of the suture through the loop that is created at the edge of the muscle (▶ Fig. 4.10a):

a) If a rectus muscle plication is planned, the suture is placed to imbricate the muscle similarly to a resection but without clamping or cauterizing the muscle at the resection site (▶ Fig. 4.19), as one purpose of performing a plication is to preserve the anterior ciliary circulation.

b) For a plication, the needles are passed partial thickness at the insertion, entering the sclera just adjacent to the poles of the insertion (▶ Fig. 4.20). The suture is tied with a 3–1–1 throw square knot as follows: first, the posterior muscle is advanced while grasping the eye near the limbus with toothed forceps and rotating the eye toward the muscle. The first 3-throw tie is held with an empty needle holder by the assistant with the muscle

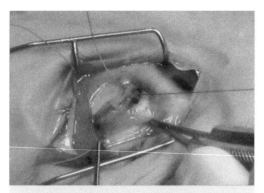

Fig. 4.20 For a plication, the needles are passed partial thickness at the poles of the insertion, entering the sclera just adjacent to the poles.

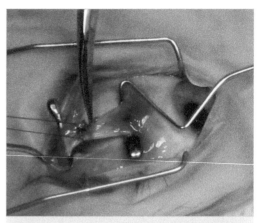

Fig. 4.21 The marked resection site has been cauterized and the muscle imbricated posterior to the mark. The sutures are held taut with the Jameson hook, and the muscle is resected with small consecutive snips.

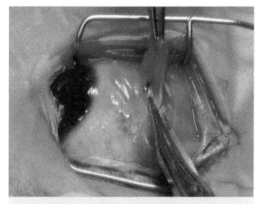

Fig. 4.22 After resection of the rectus muscle, the stump of muscle is grasped with toothed forceps, and blunt Westcott scissors are used to disinsert the stump with consecutive small snips flush to the sclera.

securely plicated, until the first 1-throw tie is ready to tighten.

5. The sutures are then gathered and held taut between the thumb and forefinger while the same hand holds the Jameson hook between the forefinger and middle finger.

6. Blunt Westcott scissors are used to resect the muscle with consecutive small snips (▶ Fig. 4.21). The sutures should not be held excessively taut to avoid a sudden movement when the muscle is completely resected.

7. The sutures are then released.

8. The stump of muscle at the insertion is grasped with toothed forceps, and blunt Westcott scissors are used to disinsert the stump with small consecutive snips nearly flush to the sclera

(▶ Fig. 4.22), leaving a small stump of tendon that can be securely grasped.

9. The insertion is grasped with toothed forceps and cotton-tip applicators are used to dry the insertion and identify bleeding vessels. Minimal cautery is used to cauterize the vessels, aiming for the vessels at and just anterior to the insertion and avoiding cautery posterior to the insertion where the sclera is thinner.

10. The ends of the suture are pulled up to identify the poles of the muscles with their respective needles. One needle is loaded on a needle holder near its center. The insertion is securely grasped with toothed forceps. The tip of the needle is then oriented tangential to and pointed slightly away from the sclera. The needle is engaged partial thickness in the sclera at one pole of the original insertion or with vertical displacement if planned for pattern strabismus or a small vertical deviation. The needle may enter the sclera nearly at the base of the small ridge at the original insertion and is then carefully advanced partial thickness anteriorly, ensuring that the needle is visible along the entire scleral tract without being too shallow (▶ Fig. 4.23). The path of the needle may be directed toward the center of the area anterior to the insertion or perpendicular to the insertion.

11. The above step is repeated for the opposite pole of the muscle. The assistant retracts the conjunctiva with a Stevens hook if needed.

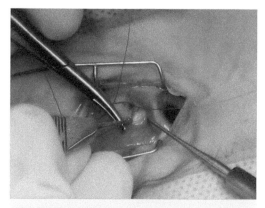

Fig. 4.23 The needle is engaged partial thickness in the sclera at one pole of the original insertion and then carefully advanced partial thickness anteriorly, ensuring that the needle is visible along the entire scleral tract without being too shallow.

12. The muscle is pulled up to the insertion using both ends of the suture. This is facilitated by rotating the globe toward the operative muscle with toothed forceps at the insertion.

13. A 3–1-1 throw square knot is tied to secure the muscle. The first 3-throw knot should be held with an empty needle holder by the assistant and only released once the first 1-throw knot is ready to tighten, to keep the resected muscle, which is usually on some degree of tension, pulled up to the original insertion. Any Tenon's capsule that becomes pulled into the knot should be released before tightening the knot.

14. Once the muscle suture is tied down, the muscle can be evaluated for central sag. If central sag is present, one end of the suture can be passed full thickness through the center of the muscle at its insertion, passing the needle from the underside of the muscle. The suture is then tied with or without a short partial-thickness scleral pass at the insertion, pulling the central portion of the muscle in line with the poles.

4.8.5 Completion of Surgery

1. Once the recessed or resected muscle is confirmed to be in good position, the suture is trimmed to leave 2 to 3 mm tails that will lie flat and not unravel.

2. The conjunctival fornix incision is reapproximated as described in Chapter 3.8.1 Fornix Incision, usually not requiring sutured closure.

4.9 Tips and Pearls

4.9.1 Before Starting Surgery

- Forced duction testing is done in eyes with a prior history of strabismus surgery or suspected extraocular restriction, but it is beneficial to become familiar with normal forced ductions by performing this procedure in all patients.
- If a unilateral recession and resection procedure is planned, the recession should be performed first, as some degree of restriction occurs following rectus muscle resections, altering free rotation of the globe.
- Operating on the lateral rectus muscles is thought to affect the distance alignment more than the near alignment, while operating on the medial rectus muscles affects the near alignment more than the distance alignment. This is considered when planning both unilateral and bilateral strabismus surgery for a patient with distance–near disparity.
- ▶ Table 4.1 is a starting point for horizontal rectus muscle recessions and resections, but there are variations in how the table can be used, and it may be adjusted based on the surgeon's own techniques and outcomes. For example, in patients with lateral gaze incomitance undergoing unilateral surgery, the amount of surgery on the medial and lateral rectus muscles can be based on the muscle's field of action and the deviations measured in lateral gazes, rather than solely using the table numbers for the primary gaze deviation.

4.9.2 Use of Muscle Hooks and Forceps

- A Stevens hook is used by the assistant throughout the surgery to retract conjunctiva and Tenon's capsule for adequate exposure of the operative muscles and sclera. The hook is usually rotated to be as flat as possible on the eye.
- For some surgeons, locking toothed forceps may lessen the need for a trained surgical assistant.
- Recall the spiral of Tillaux and avoid attempting to hook the lateral, inferior, and superior rectus muscles too far posteriorly, which can result in inadvertent hooking of an oblique muscle or tendon.
- Using the Guyton hook can help maintain a small conjunctival incision by easily gathering the width of the muscle in the elbow of the hook.

4.9.3 Imbricating the Muscle

- Tenon's capsule in young children is robust and requires careful attention to avoid its incorporation into suture passes on the muscle and on the sclera.
- The grooved Wright hook can be used to safely imbricate the muscle with better protection of the sclera, especially for tight rectus muscles.
- When imbricating the muscle, one method to confirm that the partial-thickness pass to the edge of the muscle is not full thickness is by carefully releasing and examining the needle while it is being passed within the muscle. If the pass is partial thickness, the needle should not move. If the pass is full thickness, the tip of the needle will tilt down toward the sclera, in which case the partial-thickness pass should be redone.
- When imbricating the muscle, the full-thickness pass to lock the suture is most safely done by passing the needle from the underside of the muscle, so that the tip of the needle is not pointed toward the globe. A Stevens hook can also be used to slightly displace the edge of the muscle away from the globe to create more room to pass the needle under the muscle. The ease of passing the needle from the underside of the muscle may depend on the position of the surgeon's hand and whether a forehanded pass or backhanded pass is needed.
- Locking the suture at the edge of the muscle is best secured by first pulling tight the segment of suture between the loop and muscle (▶ Fig. 4.10b), and then pulling the end of the suture perpendicular to the muscle fibers.

4.9.4 Disinsertion of the Muscle

- When disinserting a muscle, small consecutive snips with blunt Westcott scissors or Aebli corneal section scissors should be used to be mindful of where blades are located with every snip, thereby avoiding cutting the suture during disinsertion and also avoiding cutting into sclera, especially in patients with tight muscles which may tent the sclera when the sutures are held taut.
- If a grooved Wright hook is used to imbricate a tight rectus muscle, the Wright hook may be replaced by a Guyton hook or Jameson hook for more room during disinsertion.

4.9.5 Reinsertion of the Muscle

- The sclera where the muscle is to be reinserted should be clean and dry for optimal visualization during the partial-thickness scleral pass.
- During reinsertion of the muscle, the security of the partial-thickness scleral pass can be assessed while the tip of the needle is exiting the sclera by gently tugging on the needle perpendicular to the surface of the sclera. However, if the needle is pulled with excessive force, it may cheesewire through even a suitable scleral tract, and the pass will need to be repeated at a slightly different location.
- Some surgeons prefer to use a nonlocking needle holder to decrease the risk of scleral perforation by the swaged end of the needle. Although the swaged end is not sharp, if a locking needle holder is not in fact unlocked when quickly reloading the needle, the swaged end may be pushed into the sclera.
- As the suture is pulled through the partial-thickness scleral pass, adjacent Tenon's capsule may need to be retracted away from the suture with a small hook or forceps to keep it from being pulled into the scleral tract. If this occurs, pause pulling the suture, and release the entrapped Tenon's capsule away from the suture and scleral tract before continuing to pull the suture.
- When vertically displacing a horizontal rectus muscle for pattern strabismus, the new insertion site for the pole of the muscle closest to the original insertion is ascertained first. Then the new insertion site for the pole of the muscle furthest from the original insertion is determined by measuring the distance radially from the limbus, rather than from the insertion, especially if a large full-tendon width vertical displacement is planned.
- While the crossed-swords technique used by some surgeons maintains the broad muscle insertion and brings the sutures together after reinsertion, the requisite long scleral passes may pose a greater risk for scleral perforation. A modified technique, as described in this section, using shorter scleral passes or even parallel scleral passes that are perpendicular to the insertion can be used to securely reinsert the muscle, allowing the surgeon's hands to be comfortably positioned during this critical step.
- A double-armed 6–0 polyester nonabsorbable suture may be used for very large medial rectus recessions and also for inferior rectus recessions, which may not adhere well to the globe during healing. When using nonabsorbable suture, the

muscle should be reinserted approximately 4.0 mm posterior to the original insertion, which is incorporated into the total recession amount, to decrease the risk of the suture eroding through the conjunctiva.

4.9.6 Rectus Muscle Recessions

- During imbrication of a muscle for a recession, suture placement should be near the insertion to avoid effectively resecting the muscle, resulting in a smaller recession than intended, while still allowing room for disinsertion of the muscle without cutting the suture.
- Some surgeons do not place the central full-thickness knot when imbricating the muscle, particularly for rectus muscle recessions, as the muscle is not on tension when it is reinserted. This decreases the surgical time but may risk central sagging of the muscle. For rectus muscle resections, the muscle is on tension, and it is advised to place the central full-thickness knot.
- When performing a hangback recession, the muscle is pulled up to the insertion, and the recession distance is measured with calipers along the length of the muscle suture from the insertion. Depending on the type of scleral passes used during reinsertion, this measurement usually requires a small modification, to be approximately 0.75 mm longer than the planned distance, to achieve the planned amount of recession due to the angle at which the suture hangs the muscle back. A second technique for small to moderate recessions is to allow the muscle to hang back and tie the first 3-throw tie, then adjust the muscle position while grasping the insertion to rotate the eye away from the muscle. Once the muscle is positioned at the planned recession distance, the first 3-throw tie is securely held by the assistant with an empty needle holder, and the subsequent two 1-throw knots are tied and secured. The empty needle holder is released after the first 1-throw knot.
- If restriction of a rectus muscle is noted during forced duction testing at the start of surgery, it is useful to repeat forced duction testing intra-operatively and at the conclusion of surgery to ensure that the restriction is adequately treated.

4.9.7 Rectus Muscle Resections and Plications

- Judicious cautery is used at the resection site prior to suture placement and resection of the muscle. Excess cautery may spread, broadening the resection site, and possibly weaken the resection site before securing the muscle on suture.
- Because a resected muscle is on tension, ensure that the partial-thickness scleral passes are of adequate depth, while still visible along the scleral tract, when reinserting the muscle.
- When a rectus muscle is plicated, the anterior muscle ideally remains against the sclera under the plicated muscle. An iris spatula may be used to flatten the anterior muscle against the sclera during plication.

4.9.8 Vertical Rectus Muscle Surgery

- As previously noted, inferior rectus muscle surgery has a greater risk of overcorrection if the muscle does not properly reattach to the globe. Thus, a double armed 6–0 polyester nonabsorbable suture may be used to ensure that the muscle remains attached to the globe. When using nonabsorbable suture, the muscle should be reinserted approximately 4.0 mm posterior to the original insertion, which is incorporated into the total recession amount, to decrease the risk of the suture eroding through the conjunctiva.
- Far posterior blunt dissection with Westcott scissors over the superior and inferior rectus muscles, with awareness of the locations of the vortex veins and oblique tendon and muscle, is important to prevent postoperative changes in the eyelid position that can occur with recessions and resections. For the inferior rectus muscle, fascial attachments to the lower eyelid are dissected 15 to 18 mm posterior to the inferior rectus insertion. The risk of a change in eyelid position after vertical rectus muscle surgery may be lower in children compared to older adults.
- Dissection of the intermuscular septum during superior rectus surgery risks injury to the underlying superior oblique tendon, but the fascial connection between the superior rectus and the superior oblique should be separated for superior rectus resections and large recessions.
- During superior and inferior rectus surgery, the eyelid speculum may be removed and a small

Desmarres retractor, or one blade of a closed blade speculum, placed on the upper or lower eyelid to provide better exposure.

4.10 What to Avoid

- Tearing or creating a buttonhole in the conjunctiva.
- Uncontrolled bleeding and hematoma formation while bluntly dissecting Tenon's capsule from the muscle and the sclera anterior to the insertion.
- Inadvertently hooking and incorporating an oblique muscle or tendon into lateral, inferior, or superior rectus surgery.
- Splitting a rectus muscle with a muscle hook.
- Inadvertently cutting the suture during disinsertion or resection of the muscle; the suture can be replaced, but this is more difficult once the muscle is disinserted.
- Central sagging of the muscle after reinsertion
- A change in the eyelid position, especially with vertical rectus muscle surgery.

4.11 Complications

In addition to the complications of strabismus surgery stated in Chapter 1.11 Complications, anterior segment ischemia is a greater risk if more than two to three rectus muscles are disinserted in one eye.

4.12 Postoperative Care and Expectations

See Chapter 1.12, Postoperative Care and Expectations.

References

[1] Pineles SL, Deitz LW, Velez FG. Postoperative outcomes of patients initially overcorrected for intermittent exotropia. J AAPOS. 2011; 15(6):527–531

[2] Calhoun JH, Harley RD. Surgery for abnormal head position in congenital nystagmus. Trans Am Ophthalmol Soc. 1973; 71:70–83, discussion 84–87

[3] Del Monte MA, Archer SM. Atlas of pediatric ophthalmology and strabismus surgery. New York, NY: Churchill Livingstone; 1993

[4] Wright KW. Color Atlas of strabismus surgery: strategies and techniques, 3rd ed. New York, NY: Springer; 2007

[5] Oltra EZ, Pineles SL, Demer JL, Quan AV, Velez FG. The effect of rectus muscle recession, resection and plication on anterior segment circulation in humans. Br J Ophthalmol. 2015; 99 (4):556–560

[6] Scott WE, Drummond GT, Keech RV. Vertical offsets of horizontal recti muscles in the management of A and V pattern strabismus. Aust N Z J Ophthalmol. 1989; 17(3):281–288

[7] Guyton DL. Strabismus: history, principles, surgical anatomy, surgical options and indications. In: Gottsch JD, Stark WJ, Goldberg MF, eds. Ophthalmic Surgery, 5th ed. London: Arnold; 1999:64–72

[8] Rosenbaum AL, Santiago AP, Eds. Clinical strabismus management: principles and surgical techniques. Philadelphia, PA: Saunders Company; 1999

[9] Cestari DM, Hunter DG, Eds. Learning strabismus surgery: a case-based approach. Philadelphia, PA: Lippincott Williams & Wilkins; 2013

5 Adjustable Suture Technique

Sylvia H. Yoo

Summary

The adjustable suture technique is a debated topic amongst pediatric ophthalmologists and strabismus specialists with groups that are strong proponents for and against the use of adjustable sutures, in both children and adults. Many strabismus surgeons use adjustable sutures for select cases only.

Keywords: adjustable suture, adjustable sliding noose, clove hitch, hangback recession, traction suture

5.1 Goals

- Improve the short- and long-term outcomes of strabismus surgery by reducing undercorrections and overcorrections.
- Decrease the risk of requiring additional surgery.

5.2 Advantages

Strabismus surgery outcomes are dependent not only on the surgeon and amount of surgery, but also on the patient's potential for fusion and healing of the muscle(s). For cases that may be less predictable due to prior surgeries and abnormalities of the extraocular muscles or orbit, the adjustable suture technique is a useful option to modify the position of the muscles before healing of the surgical site. While the adjustable suture technique requires additional time in the operating room and during adjustment, the added effort may be offset if additional surgery is avoided.[1]

The adjustable sliding noose technique allows the surgeon to more easily gauge the amount of adjustment done, if needed, compared to the bowtie slipknot technique. For the bowtie slipknot technique, the muscle is reinserted, and then the muscle suture is tied in a half-bowtie, which can be untied for adjustment if needed or pulled through into a square knot to secure the position of the muscle. The bowtie slipknot technique is suitable for intraoperative adjustment of superior oblique surgery. The adjustable sliding noose technique has variations including a removable noose, which uses a clove hitch with three slip knots and can be removed from the muscle suture[2] to lessen the amount of buried suture at the conclusion of surgery. The short tag noose uses a shorter adjustable sliding noose, which is buried under the conjunctiva, so that immediate or delayed adjustment is possible.[3] For the short tag noose technique, if no adjustment is required, the buried sutures, including the short tag noose, remain untouched postoperatively. In patients with robust Tenon's capsule, isolating and adjusting the short tag noose on the muscle suture can be challenging.

5.3 Expectations

- Adjustments should be able to be performed without difficulty or significant patient discomfort.
- In the pediatric population, the adjustable suture technique can be considered in some teenage patients with topical anesthesia, but for most children, brief sedation, usually with propofol, is required.[4] If repeat sedation is required, the clinical location for adjustment depends on the surgical center and may be done in the post-anesthesia care unit or after returning to the operating room.
- Once the position of the muscle is finalized, with or without adjustment, postoperative healing should be similar to nonadjustable strabismus surgery.

5.4 Key Principles

The adjustable suture technique can be used for all four rectus muscles by performing the surgery with the patient under general anesthesia and evaluating the alignment after the patient has awoken from anesthesia. The basic principles of the hangback technique are used with placement of the muscle suture at the original insertion in most cases for both recessions and resections. All the operative rectus muscles may be placed on adjustable sutures, or one muscle may be selected for adjustable suture placement, usually the muscle on the deviating or nondominant eye, or the muscle that has been recessed. Adjustable sutures are not used for the inferior oblique muscle due to its posterior location. Adjustable sutures can be used for certain superior oblique procedures with intraoperative adjustment based on forced duction testing and fundus torsion.

Recommended instruments for performing strabismus surgery adjustments are listed in ▶ Table 5.1. An assistant is also needed during adjustments.

Table 5.1 Instruments with brief descriptions of their uses for strabismus surgery adjustments with an assistant

Locking fine needle drivers	Three needle drivers for holding the traction suture, to adjust the sliding adjustable noose, and to tie the adjustable suture
Blunt Westcott scissors	To safely trim suture
Small muscle hook	To reposition conjunctiva and suture
0.5 mm nonlocking forceps	To reposition conjunctiva
Speculum with closed leaflets	For adjustment of the superior and inferior rectus muscles, and the superior oblique tendon

5.5 Indications

Some strabismus surgeons offer the adjustable suture technique for all patients, while some reserve the adjustable suture technique for complex cases, including:

- Reoperations.
- Dysinnervation syndromes, such as Duane syndrome.
- Cranial nerve palsies.
- Restrictive strabismus.
- Orbital anomalies.

5.6 Contraindications

- Patients who are at high risk of anesthesia complications if sedation is required for adjustment.
- Patient and family preference for nonadjustable strabismus surgery.
- Patients, including teenagers, who are unlikely to tolerate adjustment with topical anesthesia, if repeat sedation is not established at the surgical center.

5.7 Preoperative Preparation

To help determine if a patient will tolerate adjustment with topical anesthesia, the technique is discussed with the patient's family and also with pediatric patients who are able to assent to surgery. The patient's tolerance of eye drop administration in the office can be assessed first. If eye drops are well-tolerated, a topical anesthetic is instilled and the conjunctiva is gently touched and moved over the sclera with a cotton-tip applicator. If this is well-tolerated by the patient, the patient may tolerate

adjustable strabismus surgery with topical anesthesia, although the sensations during adjustment are notably different. If this is not well-tolerated by the patient, or it is otherwise determined that the patient will not tolerate adjustable strabismus surgery which is otherwise indicated for the condition, a plan for repeat sedation can be discussed with the anesthesiologist preoperatively. In some cases, nonadjustable strabismus surgery may be planned instead, with the understanding that additional surgery may be needed, especially for complex cases.

5.8 Operative Technique

The conjunctival incision, isolation, and imbrication of the rectus muscle for recession or resection are described in Chapters 3 and 4. The following are the subsequent steps for adjustable suture placement using an adjustable sliding noose:

1. Once the operative muscle has been imbricated and then disinserted or resected, the ends of the muscle suture are held up to identify the poles of the muscles with their respective needles. One end is chosen and the needle loaded on a needle holder near its center. The insertion is securely grasped with toothed forceps. The tip of the needle is then oriented tangential to and pointed slightly away from the sclera. The needle is engaged partial thickness in the sclera at one pole of the original insertion or with vertical displacement if planned for pattern strabismus or a small vertical deviation. The needle may enter the sclera nearly at the base of the small ridge at the original insertion, and then carefully advanced partial thickness anteriorly, ensuring that the needle is visible along the entire scleral tract without being too shallow. The path of the needle may be directed toward the center of the area anterior to the insertion or perpendicular to the insertion.

2. The above step is repeated for the opposite pole of the muscle. The exit points of both sutures anterior to the insertion should be 1 to 2 mm apart, either by using a modified crossed-swords technique or parallel scleral passes in close proximity to each other (▶ Fig. 5.1). If the ends of the muscle suture are too widely spaced, the adjustable sliding noose will not slide easily along the muscle suture, especially when the muscle is pulled up to the insertion, such as for a resection.

3. The two ends of the muscle suture are tied together in an overhand knot using an empty needle holder (▶ Fig. 5.2), leaving ample length

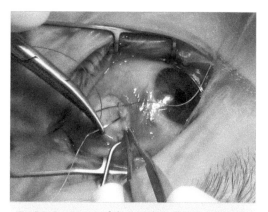

Fig. 5.1 Reinsertion of the muscle at the insertion with partial-thickness scleral passes. The exit points anterior to the insertion are in close proximity to each other with nearly parallel scleral passes.

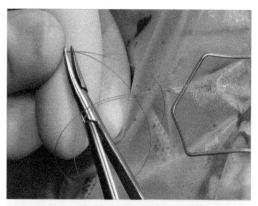

Fig. 5.2 The two ends of the muscle suture are tied together in an overhand knot using an empty needle holder.

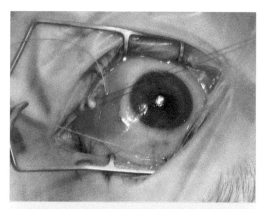

Fig. 5.3 The assistant holds the muscle suture taut across the eye with a needle holder. For placement of the adjustable sliding noose, a remnant of polyglactin suture is first tucked between the muscle suture and the insertion by the surgeon using two needle holders.

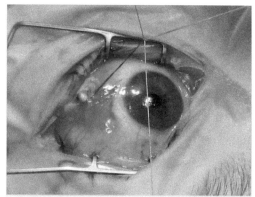

Fig. 5.4 The polyglactin suture remnant is wrapped around the muscle suture two full rotations and then tied with a 1–1 throw square knot.

of suture between the muscle and the knot for later adjustment and final tying of the suture. The tails of the suture distal to the knot should also be of adequate length to use as the adjustable sliding noose.

4. The tails are trimmed, and then the needle is trimmed off one remnant of the polyglactin suture. The assistant holds the muscle suture taut across the eye with an empty needle holder, being careful not to drag the suture on the cornea. The surgeon uses two additional empty needle holders to tuck the suture remnant between the muscle suture and insertion site (▶ Fig. 5.3), and then to wrap the suture remnant two full rotations around the muscle

suture. The assistant may hold one end of the adjustable suture to prevent it from unraveling during this step. The suture remnant is then tied with a 1–1 throw square knot (▶ Fig. 5.4) with sufficient tightness for the sliding noose to remain in position without sliding too loosely but also not excessively tight so that it is difficult to slide the noose along the muscle suture during adjustment. The assistant continues to hold the muscle suture taut. The ends of the adjustable sliding noose can be brought together by placing the two needle holders around the ends of the adjustable noose at a 90-degree angle (▶ Fig. 5.5), and then the ends are tied in an overhand knot to more easily grasp both ends of the adjustable noose during adjustment. One end of the adjustable noose is trimmed short

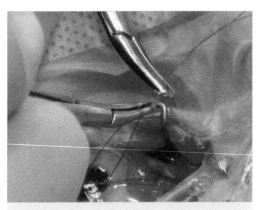

Fig. 5.5 The ends of the adjustable sliding noose on the muscle suture are brought together by placing the two needle holders around the suture at a 90-degree angle.

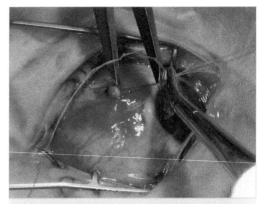

Fig. 5.6 For an adjustable rectus muscle recession, calipers set at the planned amount of recession are used to measure from the insertion, along the length of suture to determine where the adjustable sliding noose should be positioned.

and one left moderately long to easily distinguish between the adjustable sliding noose and the muscle suture during adjustment.

5. For a recession, the muscle is first pulled up to the insertion by both ends of the muscle suture. Calipers set at the planned amount of recession are used to measure from the insertion, along the length of suture toward the needles (▶ Fig. 5.6). The adjustable sliding noose is slid to the distal tip of the calipers by holding the adjustable noose with one needle holder and the muscle suture with a second needle holder (▶ Fig. 5.7). The insertion is then grasped to rotate the globe away from the muscle so that the muscle hangs back. A needle holder can also be used to pull the sutures posteriorly through the scleral tunnels if needed. The planned amount of recession is confirmed with calipers.

6. For a resection, the muscle is pulled up to the insertion, and the adjustable sliding noose is adjusted to be at or near the insertion on the muscle suture. A small amount of recession may be incorporated into the surgical plan for a resection to provide room for additional tightening during adjustment if needed.

7. Next, a single-armed polyester nonabsorbable suture, which is usually white to easily distinguish from the violet polyglactin suture, is placed on the side of the insertion and muscle suture away from the conjunctival incision, to be used as a traction suture during adjustment and to aid exposure of the adjustable sutures during adjustment (▶ Fig. 5.8). For example, for an inferiorly placed conjunctival incision, the traction suture is placed at the insertion

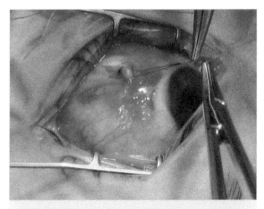

Fig. 5.7 The noose is adjusted by holding the adjustable noose with one needle holder (upper instrument in figure) and the muscle suture with a second needle holder (lower instrument in figure). In this instance, the second needle holder is holding the muscle suture distal to the adjustable noose, which is being moved proximally toward the muscle.

superior to the muscle suture with a partial-thickness pass perpendicular to the insertion while securely grasping the insertion with toothed forceps. An optional second pass of the traction suture for improved traction and exposure can be placed as follows: the ends of the muscle suture and the adjustable noose are tucked away from the sclera anterior to the insertion, where a second partial-thickness pass is placed, this time parallel to the insertion. The ends of the traction suture are gathered with the central loop if the second pass is made, and tied together in an overhand knot (▶ Fig. 5.9). The needle is trimmed.

8. Once the muscle and sutures are in good position, the conjunctival incision is reapproximated to partially cover the adjustable sutures.

9. At the conclusion of surgery, the sutures are taped with one or two 0.5-inch strips of paper tape, either on the nasal bridge for a nasally located conjunctival incision or on the temple for a temporally located conjunctival incision, after cleaning and drying the patient's skin (▶ Fig. 5.10). The sutures can be gathered onto a small area on the skin with a needle holder.

5.8.1 At the Time of Adjustment

1. Once the patient is awake and alert from anesthesia, the alignment is evaluated by cover testing or by corneal light reflex testing, at least in primary gaze and at near to determine if adjustment is needed. A topical anesthetic is instilled to help the patient open the eyes for this assessment.

2. For adjustment and trimming of the sutures, the surgeon is positioned on the side of the eye to be adjusted. The assistant helps hold the eyelid open with one or two cotton-tip applicators or gloved fingers. The assistant holds the polyester traction suture using a needle holder to retract the conjunctiva for exposure of the adjustable sutures, being careful not to drag the suture on the eyelid margin, which can cause additional discomfort, even in a sedated patient. In a patient who is awake, the patient is asked to look in the opposite direction of the operative muscle to better expose the muscle. For example, when adjusting the left medial rectus muscle, the surgeon is positioned on the patient's left side, and the patient is asked to look to left. For the left lateral rectus muscle, patient is asked to look to the right. In a sedated patient, the eye is rotated using the traction suture.

3. If the muscle needs to be recessed, the adjustable sliding noose is moved distally away from the

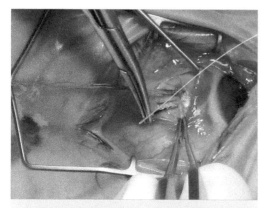

Fig. 5.8 A single-armed polyester nonabsorbable suture, which is white, is placed on the side of the insertion and muscle suture away from the conjunctival incision, to be used as a traction suture during adjustment and to aid exposure of the adjustable sutures during adjustment. In this figure, the lateral rectus has been placed on an adjustable suture through an inferotemporal conjunctival incision. The traction suture is thus placed at the insertion superior to the muscle suture, so that it can be used to retract the conjunctiva superiorly away from the adjustable suture. Also note that the violet polyglactin muscle suture and adjustable noose have already been tucked away from the sclera anterior to the insertion, where a second partial-thickness pass can placed, parallel to the insertion.

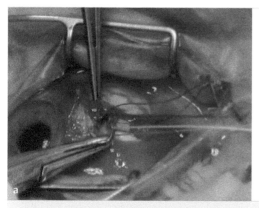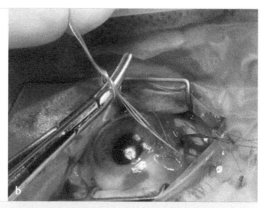

Fig. 5.9 (a) A second pass of the traction suture is placed anterior and parallel to the insertion. (b) The ends of the traction suture are gathered with the central loop and tied together in an overhand knot.

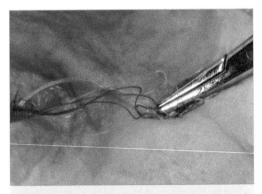

Fig. 5.10 The adjustable sutures are taped to the nasal bridge or temple after gathering the sutures onto a small area of the skin with a needle holder.

muscle using two needle holders, with the first needle holder holding the adjustable noose and the second needle holder holding both sides of the muscle suture just proximal to the adjustable noose, between the insertion and the adjustable noose. After adjustment, the traction suture can be used to rotate the eye away from the muscle to allow the muscle to hang back to the adjusted, recessed position. If the muscle needs to be advanced, the adjustable sliding noose is moved proximally toward the muscle using two needle holders, with the first needle holder holding the adjustable noose and the second needle holder holding the muscle suture just distal to the adjustable noose.

4. If the patient is awake, the alignment can be re-assessed at this time and adjustment repeated if needed. If sedation is required for adjustment, there may be rare cases when a second adjustment is needed, which is coordinated with the anesthesiologist; otherwise, adjustment is performed once.

5. Once the adjustment is complete, the muscle suture is trimmed just proximal to the overhand knot to allow ample length of suture to easily tie a 3–1–1 throw square knot over the adjustable sliding noose. Both the adjustable sliding noose and muscle suture are trimmed to leave 2 to 3 mm tails that will lie flat. The traction suture is completely removed, and the conjunctiva is gently massaged to reapproximate the incision.

5.9 Tips and Pearls

- The use of closely placed, nearly parallel needle passes for reinsertion of the muscle is an alternative to the crossed-swords technique. Although

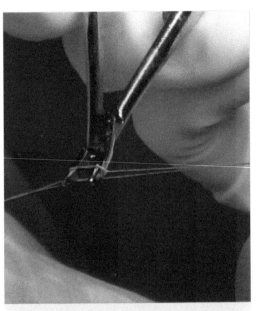

Fig. 5.11 When tying the muscle suture in an overhand knot, keep the knot loose by placing the needle holder in the knot to position it at a distance that provides ample length of suture for adjustment. To prevent the knot from sliding off the needle holder, hold one finger at the tips of the needle holder (not pictured).

the broad muscle insertion may not be maintained, adjustment with the adjustable sliding noose is performed more smoothly when the ends of the muscle suture are in close proximity to each other, and the muscle nevertheless heals well at the final insertion site.

- When tying the muscle suture in an overhand knot, maintain a loosely tied knot while pulling the ends of the suture through the loop. Then place both tips of a needle holder inside the loosely tied knot to position the knot at a distance that provides ample length of suture for adjustment and tying, before tightening the knot. Positioning of the knot is done by slowly opening and closing the needle holder while moving the knot (▶ Fig. 5.11) and while holding one finger at the tips of the needle holder to prevent the knot from sliding off the needle holder. When the loosely tied knot is at a good position, it is best to tighten the knot by using the thumb and forefinger to first grasp both lengths of the muscle suture proximally near the muscle. Then release the ends of the suture with the knot still loosely tied and slide the thumb and forefinger distally along the suture toward the knot to tighten it. This technique results in the two ends of suture from the muscle poles to be of equal length.

- For an adjustable rectus muscle recession, the muscle is pulled up to the insertion, and the adjustable sliding noose is positioned on the muscle suture at the planned recession distance measured with calipers from the insertion, along the length of the muscle suture. Due to the angle at which the suture hangs the muscle back, this measurement usually requires a small modification, to be approximately 0.75 mm longer than the planned distance, to achieve the planned amount of recession.
- If a polyester nonabsorbable suture is used on a rectus muscle for a very large recession or inferior rectus recession, a separate polyglactin suture should be used as the adjustable sliding noose. A polyester noose does not slide well on polyester suture.
- If adjustment is done while the patient is awake using a topical anesthetic, the surgeon may ask the patient whether or not she or he prefers to be made aware of the steps of adjustment and the sensations to anticipate, including pulling or pressure sensations, or the clicking sounds of the instruments.
- If the muscle needs to be recessed during adjustment, the muscle will first need to be pulled up to provide room to grasp the muscle suture just proximal to the adjustable noose, between the insertion and the adjustable noose. The patient may note a pulling sensation during this maneuver.
- A headlight is helpful to visualize the adjustable sutures and the muscle during adjustment.
- If adjustment is done under sedation, coordination of care with the anesthesiologist is key to completing the procedure efficiently and safely.

5.10 What to Avoid

Prevent any pulling of Tenon's capsule into the adjustable sliding noose during surgery and during adjustment; if this occurs, the adjustable sliding noose will not slide smoothly along the muscle suture, making adjustment more difficult.

5.11 Complications

- Slippage of the adjustable sliding noose which should then be tightened and adjusted.
- Exposure of sutures.
- Vasovagal response during adjustment.
- Some patients who may seem to be appropriate candidates for adjustment may in fact be intolerant of adjustment with topical anesthesia. Patients should be kept NPO (nothing by mouth) in the post-anesthesia care unit, in the event that repeat sedation is required to complete adjustment and trim the sutures after the alignment has been assessed.

5.12 Postoperative Care

There is a slightly higher risk of exposure of the muscle suture after adjustable strabismus surgery due to additional handling of the surrounding tissue. A topical steroid and antibiotic ointment, rather than an eye drop, may improve postoperative discomfort if this occurs.

References

[1] Leffler CT, Vaziri K, Cavuoto KM, et al. Strabismus surgery reoperation rates with adjustable and conventional sutures. Am J Ophthalmol. 2015; 160(2):385–390.e4
[2] Deschler EK, Irsch K, Guyton KL, Guyton DL. A new, removable, sliding noose for adjustable-suture strabismus surgery. J AAPOS. 2013; 17(5):524–527
[3] Nihalani BR, Whitman MC, Salgado CM, Loudon SE, Hunter DG. Short tag noose technique for optional and late suture adjustment in strabismus surgery. Arch Ophthalmol. 2009; 127(12):1584–1590
[4] Kassem A, Xue G, Gandhi NB, Tian J, Guyton DL. Adjustable suture strabismus surgery in infants and children: a 19-year experience. J AAPOS. 2018; 22(3):174–178.e1

6 Inferior Oblique Muscle Surgery

Sylvia H. Yoo

Summary

Surgery on the inferior oblique muscle involves varying degrees of weakening and, in some cases, transposition of the muscle to alter its vector force and path which normally originates at the maxillary bone and inserts on the globe near the macula.

Keywords: inferior oblique, recession, myectomy, anterior transposition, denervation and extirpation

6.1 Goals

- Resolve vertical and torsional diplopia.
- Improve an anomalous head position, which may be due to incomitant vertical strabismus caused by a unilateral trochlear nerve paresis or associated with a dissociated vertical deviation.[1]
- Improve inferior oblique overaction which may be an underlying cause of a manifest dissociated vertical deviation or associated with a large V-pattern in horizontal strabismus.

6.2 Advantages

- Treatment with inferior oblique surgery is more effective than prism glasses if torsional diplopia and significant incomitance are present.
- Patients undergoing strabismus surgery for a horizontal deviation with a large V-pattern may benefit from simultaneous inferior oblique surgery.

6.3 Expectations

- Visualization of the inferior oblique muscle with adequate exposure prior to hooking the muscle.
- Isolation of the entire inferior oblique muscle, including identification of multiple muscle bellies,[2] if present, without disrupting adjacent orbital fat or the inferotemporal vortex vein, or injury to the inferior and lateral rectus muscles.

6.4 Key Principles

- The inferior oblique muscle can undergo weakening by various degrees, or transposition, depending on the procedure performed:

  - Recession with reinsertion of the inferior oblique measured from the temporal pole of the inferior rectus insertion.
  - Myectomy can be graded from moderate to large.
  - Anterior transposition which converts the inferior oblique to a depressor.[3]
  - Denervation and extirpation, during which a large myectomy is performed and the neurofibrovascular bundle is transected, weakening the inferior oblique by the greatest amount and reserved for only severe, recurrent cases.

6.5 Indications

- Unilateral trochlear nerve (4th cranial nerve) paresis causing diplopia or ocular torticollis.
- Dissociated vertical deviation with associated inferior oblique overaction or tightness on forced duction testing.
- Inferior oblique overaction, typically associated with early onset strabismus with poor fusion.
- Large V-pattern horizontal strabismus.

6.6 Contraindications

- If multiple inferior oblique weakening procedures have been performed for persistent or recurrent overaction with vertical strabismus, an alternative approach may need to be considered to attain the desired outcome. Denervation and extirpation of the inferior oblique muscle may be considered if other options are unlikely to be effective.

6.7 Preoperative Preparation

- The superior and inferior oblique muscles are assessed for underaction or overaction on versions and ductions.
- Evaluation of fundus torsion may be performed by assessing the position of the foveal reflex with respect to the optic nerve during indirect ophthalmoscopy of each eye (▶ Fig. 6.1) while the patient fixates on a target, such as the tip of a pen, held between the condensing lens and the examiner in cooperative patients, or without fixation in younger patients.

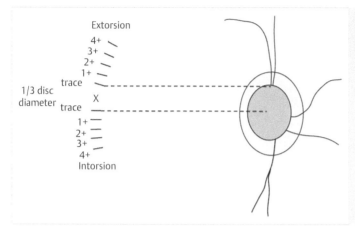

Fig. 6.1 The position of the foveal reflex with respect to the optic nerve is assessed during indirect ophthalmoscopy to evaluate for fundus torsion (left eye, inverted view).

- Torsional diplopia, if present, may be assessed with double Maddox rod testing or with Lancaster red-green testing in older children and teenagers.
- Confirmation of a suspected tight inferior oblique muscle by bilateral exaggerated traction testing, which is performed while the patient is under anesthesia before the start of surgery.

6.8 Operative Technique

6.8.1 Exaggerated Traction Testing

Evaluation of the tightness of the oblique muscles should be performed bilaterally for comparison, including in cases of unilateral oblique muscle surgery.[4]

1. After placement of an eyelid speculum, the globe is grasped with toothed forceps at the nasal limbus:
   a) To evaluate the inferior oblique muscle, the globe is retropulsed and adducted first. Then the globe is depressed and intorted, rocking the surface of the globe back and forth over the inferior oblique, which is felt as a "bump," to determine the presence of laxity or restriction (► Fig. 6.2). The tightness of the inferior oblique is compared to the tightness of the ipsilateral superior oblique tendon, as well as the tightness of the contralateral inferior oblique muscle and superior oblique tendon.
   b) To evaluate the superior oblique tendon, the globe is retropulsed and adducted first. Then the globe is elevated and extorted, rocking the surface of the globe back and forth over the superior oblique tendon. The tightness of the superior oblique is compared to the tight-

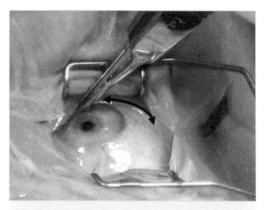

Fig. 6.2 Exaggerated traction testing of the right inferior oblique muscle is performed by grasping the globe at the 3 o'clock limbus with toothed forceps. The globe is first retropulsed and adducted, then depressed and intorted as the surface of the globe is rocked back and forth (*arrow*) over the inferior oblique muscle.

ness of the ipsilateral inferior oblique muscle, as well as the tightness of the contralateral superior oblique tendon and inferior oblique muscle.

Following creation of an inferotemporal fornix incision, as described under Chapter 3.8.1 Fornix Incision, the steps for inferior oblique muscle surgery are described below.

6.8.2 Isolation and Disinsertion of the Inferior Oblique Muscle

1. The eye continues to be grasped at the limbus, and the conjunctival incision is held open with forceps. A Stevens hook is used to isolate the lateral rectus muscle with the handle nearly

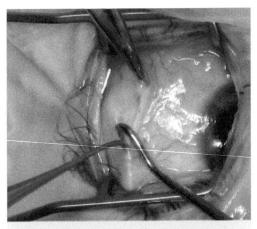

Fig. 6.3 A Jameson hook is placed on the lateral rectus muscle.

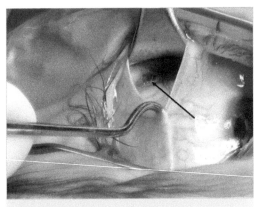

Fig. 6.4 A small Desmarres retractor retracts the conjunctiva and Tenon's capsule inferotemporally to identify the pink inferior oblique muscle (*arrow*).

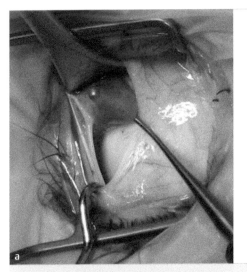

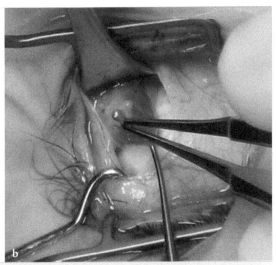

Fig. 6.5 **(a)** A Stevens hook hooks the inferior oblique which is pulled forward. **(b)** The surrounding Tenon's capsule is carefully unhooked with toothed forceps.

perpendicular to the insertion, keeping in mind the approximate location of the insertion from the limbus. Once the muscle is securely hooked, the assistant can release the forceps from the limbus, while keeping the conjunctival incision open with forceps.

2. A Jameson hook then hooks the lateral rectus muscle by placing the hook just posterior to the small hook, which is then removed (▶ Fig. 6.3). The Jameson hook is held by the assistant to provide traction and to slightly displace the lateral rectus away from the inferior oblique during surgery. Alternatively, a 4–0 silk suture can be placed under the lateral rectus using a Gass hook.

3. A small Desmarres or Conway retractor is placed in the inferotemporal conjunctival incision to retract the conjunctiva and Tenon's capsule inferotemporally. Posteriorly, the pink inferior oblique muscle can be visualized and will appear adherent to the overlying retracted tissue and not in contact with the globe (▶ Fig. 6.4). The inferotemporal vortex vein may be visible near the posterior border of the inferior oblique, just temporal to the inferior rectus and should be avoided during subsequent steps.

4. A Stevens hook is used to hook the inferior oblique from posterior to anterior, and the inferior oblique is pulled forward (▶ Fig. 6.5a). The

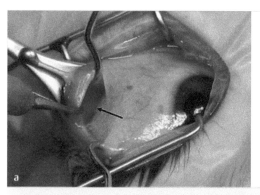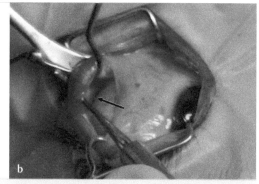

Fig. 6.6 The two hooks on the inferior oblique are slightly separated to examine the area (*arrow*) bordered by the temporal and nasal aspects of the inferior oblique muscle and the sclera in the inferotemporal quadrant. **(a)** This area which should *not* be pink and **(b)** should be white if the entire inferior oblique has been hooked.

surrounding Tenon's capsule is carefully unhooked with toothed forceps (▶ Fig. 6.5b), so that only the inferior oblique muscle remains on the hook, and the tip of the small hook can be exposed between the muscle and the connective tissue without orbital fat exposure.

5. The inferior oblique is hooked with a Jameson hook adjacent to the Stevens hook, and the hooks are slightly separated to examine the space bordered by the temporal and nasal aspects of the inferior oblique muscle and the sclera in the inferotemporal quadrant (▶ Fig. 6.6). This area should *not* appear pink as shown in ▶ Fig. 6.6a and should be white as shown in ▶ Fig. 6.6b to indicate that the entire inferior oblique has been hooked. If this area is pink, the Jameson hook is kept in place, and the Stevens hook is used to hook the remaining portion of the inferior oblique muscle, which is rejoined with the previously hooked portion of the muscle, and steps 4 and 5 are repeated.

6. Once the inferior oblique is confirmed to be entirely hooked, the Stevens hook is removed and the surrounding fascia is bluntly dissected from the muscle both nasally and temporally with blunt Westcott scissors (▶ Fig. 6.7).

7. The inferior oblique is then clamped near its insertion with one click of a small straight clamp, allowing room to be able to visualize the muscle at its insertion and for blunt Westcott scissors to be used to disinsert the muscle. Both tips of the clamp must be visualized around the muscle before securing the clamp (▶ Fig. 6.8).

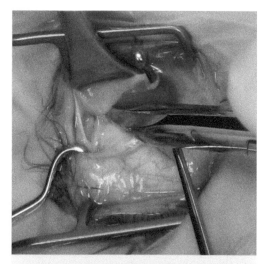

Fig. 6.7 Once the entire inferior oblique is hooked, the surrounding fascia is bluntly dissected from the muscle with blunt Westcott scissors. In this figure, the Westcott scissors are bluntly dissecting the temporal aspect of the inferior oblique toward the lateral rectus muscle.

8. The inferior oblique muscle can be first strummed at its insertion with closed blades of the blunt Westcott scissors for tactile confirmation of its location. The inferior oblique is then disinserted without excessive traction on the muscle, using small consecutive snips to be certain of the location of the scissors nearly flush to the sclera (▶ Fig. 6.9). Once the inferior oblique is disinserted, additional fascial attachments can be bluntly dissected more nasally.

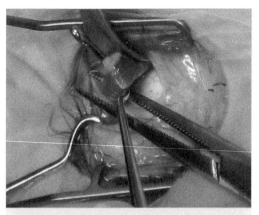

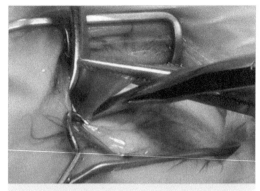

Fig. 6.9 The inferior oblique is disinserted using small consecutive snips nearly flush to the sclera.

Fig. 6.8 The inferior oblique is clamped near its insertion with a small straight clamp, allowing room for blunt Westcott scissors to disinsert the muscle. Both tips of the clamp must be visualized around the muscle before securing the clamp.

6.8.3 Inferior Oblique Recession or Anterior Transposition

1. For an inferior oblique recession or anterior transposition, a 6–0 double-armed Vicryl suture is more safely placed *after* the inferior oblique is clamped and disinserted. Each end of the suture is passed partial thickness through the width of the muscle to either edge of the muscle, followed by a full-thickness pass including one-fourth to one-third of the muscle width which is then locked by passing the end of the suture through the loop that is created at the edge of the muscle. A central knot is not necessary for the inferior oblique muscle, as the muscle is not on tension and can be reinserted with little to no risk of central sag. The clamp is then removed, and the clamped segment of muscle will reperfuse.
2. Exaggerated traction testing of the inferior oblique muscle is then repeated to confirm that the entire inferior oblique has been disinserted. As the globe is intorted, there should no longer be a "bump" felt over the inferior oblique muscle.
3. The inferior rectus muscle is then hooked with a Stevens hook followed by a Jameson hook through the inferotemporal fornix incision, and the temporal pole of the inferior rectus insertion is identified:
   a) For an anterior transposition, the inferior oblique can be reinserted just temporal to the temporal pole of the inferior rectus insertion.

b) For a recession, the muscle can be reinserted 2 mm temporal and 2 to 3 mm posterior to the temporal aspect of the inferior rectus insertion which is marked with calipers and a marking pen. Reinsertion 2 mm temporal and 3 mm posterior to the inferior rectus insertion is a recession, while reinsertion 2 mm temporal and 2 mm posterior to the inferior rectus insertion slightly anteriorizes the inferior oblique (▶ Fig. 6.10).
4. The inferior oblique is reinserted with adjacent partial-thickness needle passes at the selected insertion site (▶ Fig. 6.11a), maintaining the approximate path of the inferior oblique muscle. Relatively short passes of adequate depth will securely reattach the inferior oblique muscle.
5. Once the muscle is confirmed to be in good position (▶ Fig. 6.11b), the suture is tied with a 3–1–1 throw square knot and trimmed to leave 2 to 3 mm tails that will lie flat and not unravel.
6. The conjunctival incision can then be reapproximated.

6.8.4 Inferior Oblique Myectomy

1. For an inferior oblique myectomy, a second small curved or straight clamp is used to cross-clamp the disinserted inferior oblique muscle with care to avoid cross-clamping in an area where there is adjacent orbital fat visible, sometimes seen more nasally where the muscle becomes larger in cross-section. The amount of myectomy is determined by the preoperative measurements, as well as exaggerated traction testing of the oblique muscles.

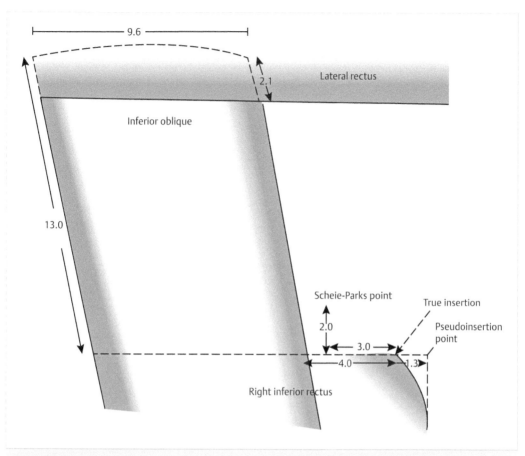

Fig. 6.10 The anatomy of the inferior oblique muscle in relation to the inferior rectus insertion determines the site of reinsertion for an inferior oblique recession or anterior transposition.

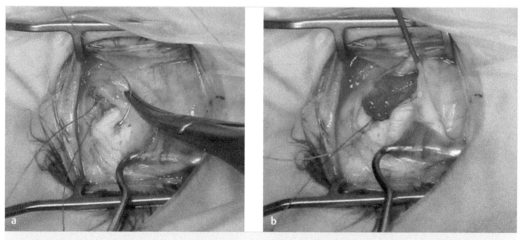

Fig. 6.11 **(a)** For an inferior oblique recession, the inferior rectus is hooked with a Jameson hook, and the muscle is reinserted with partial-thickness scleral passes at the marked location which is measured from the temporal pole of the inferior rectus insertion. **(b)** The muscle is pulled up to the new insertion site, and the suture is tied and trimmed.

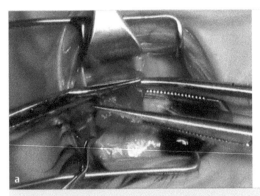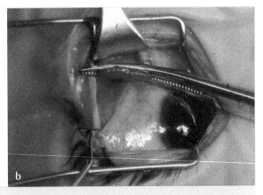

Fig. 6.12 **(a)** For an inferior oblique myectomy, the muscle is cross-clamped and then transected near the second clamp, **(b)** leaving a small stump for generous cautery to be applied.

2. The muscle is then transected near the second clamp (▶ Fig. 6.12a), leaving a small stump for generous cautery to be applied (▶ Fig. 6.12b). The stump is then cauterized with bipolar cautery.
3. The remaining clamp is slowly removed to ensure that adequate hemostasis has been achieved, and the muscle is allowed to retract through the Tenon's capsule opening.
4. Exaggerated traction testing of the inferior oblique muscle is repeated at this time to confirm that the entire inferior oblique has been disinserted. As the globe is intorted, there should no longer be a "bump" felt over the inferior oblique muscle.
5. The conjunctival incision can then be reapproximated.

6.8.5 Inferior Oblique Denervation and Extirpation

1. Once the inferior oblique is disinserted and held with the small clamp, additional blunt dissection of the surrounding fascia nasally, toward the origin of the muscle, is performed. For greater inferior exposure, the eyelid speculum may be removed and only a Desmarres retractor used to retract both the lower eyelid and the inferior conjunctiva. The inferior rectus is also hooked to elevate the globe.
2. The neurofibrovascular bundle (NVB) is located posterior and temporal to the area of fusiform enlargement of the inferior oblique. It can be strummed with a Stevens hook and then hooked to separate it from the muscle and Tenon's capsule. A second Stevens hook is positioned in the opposite direction.
3. A cellulose sponge is placed under the NVB and muscle to protect the adjacent sclera, and bipolar

cautery is carefully used to cauterize and transect the NVB. Alternatively, the NVB is clamped with a small clamp and then transected with cautery between the muscle and clamp, with additional cautery to the NVB stump before releasing into the Tenon's capsule opening.
4. Once the NVB is transected, the inferior oblique will release and become accessible further toward its origin, and additional dissection of the surrounding fascia is carefully performed.
5. A second small clamp is used to cross-clamp the inferior oblique muscle as far toward its origin as possible, with care to avoid inclusion of adjacent orbital fat. The muscle is then transected near the second clamp, leaving a small stump for generous cautery to be applied. The stump is then cauterized with bipolar cautery.
6. The second clamp is slowly removed to ensure that adequate hemostasis has been achieved, and the muscle is allowed to retract through the Tenon's capsule opening.
7. Exaggerated traction testing of the inferior oblique muscle is repeated to confirm that the entire inferior oblique has been disinserted. As the globe is intorted, there should no longer be a "bump" felt over the inferior oblique muscle.
8. The conjunctival incision can then be reapproximated.

6.9 Tips and Pearls

- The approach to unilateral trochlear nerve paresis is surgeon-dependent. Some surgeons weaken the ipsilateral inferior oblique muscle as first-line surgical treatment. Other surgeons tighten the affected superior oblique tendon, as described in Chapter 7.8.4 Superior Oblique Tuck, as first-line surgical treatment.

- A headlight is helpful but not required to visualize the more posteriorly located inferior oblique muscle.
- Isolation of the entire inferior oblique muscle is confirmed by two methods:
  - An area of white tissue bordered by the nasal and temporal aspects of the inferior oblique muscle and the sclera during isolation of the muscle with two hooks.
  - Repeat exaggerated traction testing following disinsertion.
- During denervation and extirpation of the inferior oblique muscle, avoid placing excessive traction on the NVB to decrease the risk of damage to the ciliary ganglion.
- Following inferior oblique surgery, the lateral and inferior rectus muscles are confirmed to be intact with a small hook before reapproximating the conjunctival incision.
- Surgery on the inferior oblique muscles does not significantly alter the horizontal alignment in primary gaze. Thus, a patient with a V-pattern exotropia with inferior oblique overaction should undergo strabismus surgery on the horizontal rectus muscles based on the primary gaze deviation in addition to inferior oblique weakening to treat the strabismus.

6.10 What to Avoid

- Avoid excessive manipulation and dissection around the inferior oblique muscle, which may lead to:
  - Excessive bleeding, especially with vortex vein injury.
  - Orbital fat exposure.
  - Scarring.
- Avoid blind hooking of the inferior oblique muscle.
- During disinsertion of the inferior oblique muscle, avoid excessive traction on the muscle, given that it inserts at the level of the macula.

6.11 Complications

- Orbital fat adherence due to violation of Tenon's capsule posteriorly.
- Be aware of the risk of anti-elevation following anterior transposition of the inferior oblique muscle,[5] which can be avoided by ensuring that the posterior fibers of the inferior oblique are reinserted posterior to the inferior rectus insertion,[6] unless anti-elevation is the goal of surgery in cases of recurrent dissociated vertical deviations with inferior oblique overaction. Anti-elevation occurs due to tethering of the posterior fibers of the inferior oblique muscle by the NVB, which effectively becomes an ancillary origin of the muscle when it is truly anteriorized by reinsertion anterior to the inferior rectus insertion.[7]
- Unmasking of bilateral superior oblique paresis or bilateral inferior oblique overaction can occur when unilateral surgery is performed due to marked asymmetry of the measurements, resulting in the preoperative appearance of a unilateral abnormality. Bilateral superior oblique paresis is suspected in patients who have more than 10 to 12 degrees of extorsion on double Maddox rod testing, alternating hypertropia, large esotropia in downgaze often resulting in a chin down head position, and bilateral fundus extorsion.

6.12 Postoperative Care and Expectations

- Following inferior oblique surgery, patients with significant astigmatism should be refracted postoperatively to account for a change in the astigmatism axis.[8]

References

[1] Santiago AP, Rosenbaum AL. Dissociated vertical deviation and head tilts. J AAPOS. 1998; 2(1):5–11

[2] De Angelis D, Makar I, Kraft SP. Anatomic variations of the inferior oblique muscle: a potential cause of failed inferior oblique weakening surgery. Am J Ophthalmol. 1999; 128(4): 485–488

[3] Stager DR, Jr, Beauchamp GR, Wright WW, Felius J, Stager D, Sr. Anterior and nasal transposition of the inferior oblique muscles. J AAPOS. 2003; 7(3):167–173

[4] Guyton DL. Exaggerated traction test for the oblique muscles. Ophthalmology. 1981; 88(10):1035–1040

[5] Kushner BJ. Restriction of elevation in abduction after inferior oblique anteriorization. J AAPOS. 1997; 1(1):55–62

[6] Wright KW. Color atlas of strabismus surgery: strategies and techniques, 3rd ed. New York, NY: Springer; 2007

[7] Stager DR. Costenbader lecture. Anatomy and surgery of the inferior oblique muscle: recent findings. J AAPOS. 2001; 5(4): 203–208

[8] Kushner BJ. Strabismus: practical pearls you won't find in textbooks. Cham, Switzerland: Springer; 2017

7 Superior Oblique Surgery

Catherine S. Choi and Sylvia H. Yoo

Summary
Surgery on the superior oblique tendon includes both weakening and tightening procedures to address superior oblique abnormalities resulting in incomitant cyclovertical deviations, A-pattern strabismus, and torsional diplopia.

Keywords: ocular torticollis, trochlear nerve paresis, Brown syndrome, A-pattern, tenotomy, suture spacer, superior oblique tuck, Harada-Ito procedure

7.1 Goals

- Improve ocular torticollis due to incomitant cyclovertical strabismus.
- Improve diplopia caused by superior oblique abnormalities, including trochlear nerve (4th cranial nerve) paresis and Brown syndrome.
- Improve A-pattern strabismus associated with superior oblique overaction.

7.2 Advantages

- Treatment with superior oblique surgery is often more effective than prism glasses due to the presence of torsional diplopia and incomitance from superior oblique dysfunction.
- Patients undergoing strabismus surgery for a horizontal deviation with a large A-pattern may benefit from simultaneous superior oblique surgery.

7.3 Expectations

- Long-term resolution of diplopia including torsional diplopia.
- Ability to resolve residual diplopia with prisms.
- Improvement of ocular torticollis.
- Improvement of A-pattern strabismus.

7.4 Key Principles

- The superior oblique muscle and tendon have an unusual course in comparison to the other extraocular muscles, with significant variability in morphology, including reported absence in some patients.[1]

- The anterior fibers of the muscle primarily intort the eye, while the posterior fibers primarily depress the eye. Procedures such as the Harada-Ito procedure take advantage of the compartmentalized functions of the tendon to target the torsional function of the anterior fibers.
- The superior oblique muscle also has a tertiary function of abduction, so that patients with bilateral superior oblique palsies present with esotropia in downgaze, resulting in a V-pattern esotropia.

7.5 Indications

- Superior oblique weakening procedures:
  - Superior oblique tenotomy:
    - Superior oblique overaction causing A-pattern strabismus, hypotropia in primary gaze, or ocular torticollis (head tilt).
    - Not recommended for Brown syndrome due to risk of iatrogenic superior oblique paresis.[2]
  - Superior oblique spacer:
    - Brown syndrome causing hypotropia in primary gaze, significant ocular torticollis (chin up), and diplopia.
    - Superior oblique overaction causing A-pattern strabismus, hypotropia in primary gaze, or ocular torticollis (head tilt), especially if normal stereoacuity is present.
- Superior oblique tightening procedures:
  - Superior oblique tuck:
    - Superior oblique weakness due to unilateral trochlear nerve (4th cranial nerve) paresis resulting in ocular torticollis (head tilt or head turn), hypertropia, and diplopia.
    - May be considered bilaterally for bilateral trochlear nerve paresis if a very large esotropia is present in downgaze.
  - Harada-Ito procedure:
    - Bilateral superior oblique weakness due to bilateral trochlear nerve paresis with primarily torsional diplopia, alternating hypertropia in lateral gazes, and ocular torticollis (chin down).
    - If the bilateral trochlear nerve paresis is significantly asymmetric, resulting in both torsional and vertical diplopia, Harada-Ito procedure may be performed on the less affected eye, and a superior oblique tuck performed on the more severely affected eye.

7.6 Contraindications

- Superior oblique tenotomy is not recommended in patients with normal stereoacuity, such as those with Brown syndrome and intermittent A-pattern exotropia, due to a greater risk of developing iatrogenic superior oblique paresis, resulting in torsional diplopia and ocular torticollis.

7.7 Preoperative Preparation

- Evaluation of fundus torsion may be performed by assessing the position of the foveal reflex with respect to the optic nerve during indirect ophthalmoscopy of each eye (▶ Fig. 6.1 in Chapter 6) while the patient fixates on a target, such as the tip of a pen, held between the condensing lens and the examiner in cooperative patients, or without fixation in younger patients.
- For cooperative older children and teenagers, measurements of torsion with double Maddox rod testing or Lancaster red-green testing are done during the preoperative evaluation of patients with superior oblique abnormalities and diplopia.

7.8 Operative Technique

7.8.1 Exaggerated Traction Testing[3]

Evaluation of the tightness of the oblique muscles should be performed bilaterally for comparison, including in cases of unilateral oblique muscle surgery.

1. After placement of an eyelid speculum, the globe is grasped with toothed forceps at the nasal limbus.
    a) To evaluate the superior oblique tendon, the globe is retropulsed and adducted first. Then the globe is elevated and extorted, rocking the surface of the globe back and forth over the superior oblique tendon. The tightness of the superior oblique is compared to the tightness of the ipsilateral inferior oblique muscle, as well as the tightness of the contralateral superior oblique tendon and inferior oblique muscle.
    b) To evaluate the inferior oblique muscle, the globe is retropulsed and adducted first. Then the globe is depressed and intorted, rocking the surface of the globe back and forth over

the inferior oblique, which is felt as a "bump," to determine the presence of laxity or restriction (▶ Fig. 6.2 in Chapter 6). The tightness of the inferior oblique is compared to the tightness of the ipsilateral superior oblique tendon, as well as the tightness of the contralateral inferior oblique muscle and superior oblique tendon.

A superonasal or superotemporal fornix incision, as described in Chapter 3.8.1 Fornix Incision, may be used for superior oblique surgery, depending on the procedure performed and the surgeon's preference.

7.8.2 Superior Oblique Tenotomy

1. A fornix incision is made in the superotemporal quadrant using blunt Westcott scissors, approximately 8 mm posterior to the limbus.
2. The superior rectus muscle is isolated first with a Stevens hook, and then with a Jameson hook, which is swept toward the limbus to ensure that the entire width of the muscle has been isolated.
3. A Stevens hook is used to reflect the conjunctiva over the bulb of the Jameson hook.
4. Blunt Westcott scissors are used to make a small incision in the intermuscular septum at the bulb of the Jameson hook, and a Stevens hook is inserted in the opening to perform a pole test to confirm that the entire width of the superior rectus muscle has been hooked.
5. A small Desmarres retractor is then placed in the conjunctival incision and positioned to expose the nasal aspect of the superior rectus muscle.
6. The Jameson hook is used to depress the eye and also displace the superior rectus temporally, and the Desmarres retractor is positioned for exposure of the nasal aspect of the superior oblique tendon just adjacent to and under the superior rectus muscle. The eyelid speculum may be removed at this time.
7. A Stevens hook, with its tip pointed nasally, is swept posteriorly along the nasal border of the superior rectus muscle to the posterior margin of the superior oblique tendon which is isolated onto the Stevens hook.
8. The Tenon's capsule surrounding the tendon is carefully dissected with 0.3-mm toothed forceps and Westcott scissors. A second Stevens hook is passed under the superior oblique tendon in the opposite direction of the first Stevens hook.

9. Blunt Westcott scissors are then used to incise the tendon between the two Stevens hooks for a complete tenotomy.
10. All of the instruments are removed, and exaggerated traction testing is repeated to confirm that the superior oblique is free following complete tenotomy. Any residual tension suggests an incomplete tenotomy, which should prompt the surgeon to repeat the above procedure and explore for additional fibers of the superior oblique tendon that may have been overlooked.
11. The conjunctival incision is reapproximated, usually not requiring sutured closure.

7.8.3 Superior Oblique Tenotomy with Suture Spacer

1. Indirect ophthalmoscopy after pupillary dilation may be performed to evaluate fundus torsion for comparison during intraoperative adjustment.
2. A fornix incision is made in the superonasal quadrant using blunt Westcott scissors.
3. The superior rectus muscle is isolated with a Stevens hook, followed by a Jameson hook.
4. A Stevens hook is used to drape the conjunctiva over the bulb of the Jameson hook.
5. Blunt Westcott scissors are used to make an incision in the intermuscular septum just under the bulb of the Jameson hook, and a Stevens hook is inserted in the opening to perform a pole test to confirm that the entire width of the superior rectus muscle has been hooked.
6. A small Desmarres retractor is then placed in the conjunctival incision to expose the nasal aspect of the superior rectus muscle.
7. The Jameson hook is used to depress the eye and also displace the superior rectus temporally, and the Desmarres retractor is positioned for exposure of the nasal aspect of the superior oblique tendon just adjacent to and under the superior rectus muscle. The eyelid speculum may be removed at this time.
8. A Stevens hook, with its tip pointed nasally, is swept posteriorly along the nasal border of the superior rectus muscle to the posterior margin of the superior oblique tendon which is isolated onto the hook.
9. The Tenon's capsule surrounding the tendon is carefully dissected with 0.3-mm toothed forceps and Westcott scissors. A Jameson hook is passed under the superior oblique tendon in the opposite direction of the Stevens hook. The

Jameson hook on the superior rectus muscle is then used to replace the Stevens hook on the superior oblique tendon.
10. The superior oblique tendon is held taut by the two Jameson hooks.
11. A 6–0 double-armed nonabsorbable polyester suture is secured on the temporal aspect of the superior oblique tendon just nasal to the superior rectus muscle with a central full-thickness 2–1 throw square knot. One end of the suture is wrapped from the surface of the tendon, around and under the tendon, emerging to the surface again via a full-thickness pass at one edge of the tendon. The other end of the suture is wrapped in the opposite direction, around and under the tendon, emerging to the surface again with a full-thickness pass at the opposite edge of the tendon.
12. Both needles are then passed through the nasal aspect of the tendon from the underside of the tendon, approximately 4 to 7 mm from the temporal knot. The ends of the suture at the nasal aspect of the tendon are tied in an overhand knot, leaving ample length of suture between the tendon and the knot, and the needles are trimmed (▶ Fig. 7.1).
13. Using two needle holders, an adjustable sliding noose using a segment of polyglactin suture without a needle is placed around the nasal ends of the suture spacer, which is held taut by the assistant with a needle holder, with two full turns and a 1–1 throw square knot. The ends of the adjustable sliding noose are tied together with an overhand knot, and the sliding noose is then adjusted for the suture spacer to be completely lax between the nasal and temporal tendon. A Stevens hook can be used to pull the slack of the suture between the temporal and nasal aspects of the tendon.
14. A remnant of single-armed 6–0 polyester suture is placed on the tendon just temporal to the nasal passes of the suture spacer. This suture is used as a traction suture to access the adjustable sutures and tendon during adjustment. This suture is secured on the tendon with a central full-thickness knot, pulling the suture more than halfway through the tendon before tying the knot. The long end of the suture is wrapped around the tendon and tied again, then wrapped in the opposite direction and tied a third time. The tails are trimmed to be asymmetric with one short tail and one long tail, for the traction suture to be easily differentiated from the suture spacer.

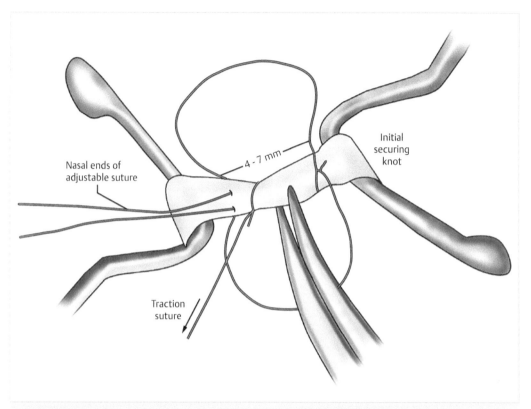

Nasal ends of
adjustable suture

4 - 7 mm

Initial
securing
knot

Traction
suture

Fig. 7.1 Placement of the adjustable superior oblique suture spacer prior to transection of the tendon. Once the tendon is transected, the suture spacer will bridge the cut ends of the suture.

15. Once the suture spacer is in place and on maximum slack, the tendon is transected between the temporal knot of the suture spacer and the traction suture nasally. Extra care is taken to avoid cutting the suture spacer.
16. Exaggerated traction testing is repeated to confirm that the entire tendon has been transected. Then the adjustable sliding noose on the suture spacer is adjusted to leave a 4 to 8 mm gap between the cut ends of the tendon, depending on the preoperative examination and initial exaggerated traction testing.
17. The Jameson hooks and small Desmarres retractor are removed, and exaggerated traction testing is repeated in both eyes for comparison. If adjustment is needed, the Desmarres retractor and Jameson hooks are replaced by means of the traction suture, and the adjustable sliding noose is adjusted on the suture spacer. If the suture spacer is adjusted for greater weakening, a Stevens hook is used to pull the slack between the cut ends of the tendon.
18. Once the suture is adjusted, exaggerated traction testing is performed again, and Step 17 is repeated until traction testing in the operative eye is similar to that in the fellow eye, aiming for a small undercorrection. Fundus torsion may also be evaluated by indirect ophthalmoscopy to help finalize the position of the suture spacer.
19. Once the spacing between the cut ends of the tendon is finalized, the suture spacer is trimmed near the overhand knot and tied in a 3–1–1 throw square knot over the polyglactin adjustable noose.
20. The ends of the suture spacer, the adjustable sliding noose, which is absorbable, and the traction suture are all trimmed.
21. The hooks and Desmarres retractor are removed, and the conjunctival incision is reapproximated, usually not requiring sutured closure.

7.8.4 Superior Oblique Tuck

1. A fornix incision is made in the superotemporal quadrant using blunt Westcott scissors, approximately 8 mm posterior to the limbus.

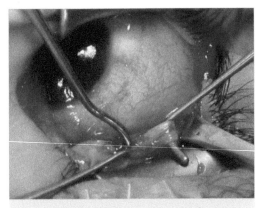

Fig. 7.2 The temporal superior oblique tendon on a Stevens hook after blunt dissection is performed.

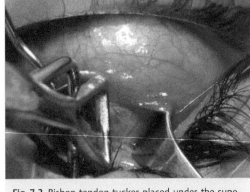

Fig. 7.3 Bishop tendon tucker placed under the superior oblique tendon.

2. The superior rectus muscle is isolated with a Stevens hook, and then with a Jameson hook, which is swept toward the limbus to ensure that the entire width of the muscle has been isolated.

3. A Stevens hook is used to reflect the conjunctiva over the bulb of the Jameson hook.

4. Blunt Westcott scissors are used to make an incision in the intermuscular septum at the bulb of the Jameson hook, and a Stevens hook is inserted in the opening to perform a pole test to confirm that the entire width of the superior rectus muscle has been isolated.

5. Two Stevens hooks are used to tent the overlying conjunctiva, and the check ligaments and Tenon's capsule overlying the superior rectus are carefully dissected with Westcott scissors.

6. A small Desmarres retractor is used to replace the Stevens hooks and positioned superotemporally.

7. The Jameson hook on the superior rectus muscle is used to displace the muscle nasally, and the eyelid speculum may be removed at this time.

8. A Stevens hook, with its tip pointed nasally, is swept posteriorly along the temporal border of the superior rectus muscle to the posterior margin of the white fibers of the superior oblique tendon, which is isolated onto the hook (▶ Fig. 7.2), with care to hook the entire tendon but avoiding the superotemporal vortex vein. The distal tendon is carefully cleared of surrounding connective tissue with blunt dissection.

9. The Stevens hook is replaced by the hook on the Bishop tendon tucker, which is adjusted until the slack in the tendon is tightened. There should be adequate tension on the tendon so

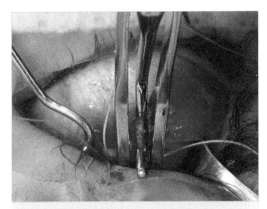

Fig. 7.4 Use of 5–0 double-armed polyester suture to tuck the tendon in a double-mattress fashion.

that the Bishop tendon tucker cannot be easily lifted off the sclera (▶ Fig. 7.3).

10. A 5–0 double-armed nonabsorbable polyester suture is used to secure the tucked tendon at its base, using a double-mattress suturing technique (▶ Fig. 7.4). A 3–1 throw bowtie slipknot is tied, and all the hooks and the Bishop tendon tucker are removed.

11. Saunder's forced duction testing[4] is performed by grasping the globe at the inferotemporal limbus and rotating the eye in an elevated and adducted position. Resistance should be felt when the inferior limbus reaches the medial canthus (Saunder's line), which confirms adequate tightening of the superior oblique tendon:

a) If the globe can be easily elevated past the Saunder's line, the superior oblique tendon should be tucked further.

b) If there is significant resistance, preventing elevation of the globe to the Saunder's line, the superior oblique tendon is too tight and at risk of causing an iatrogenic Brown syndrome, and the tuck should be relaxed.

c) If the amount of tuck requires adjustment based on Saunder's forced duction testing, the Jameson hook is used to hook the superior rectus muscle, and the Desmarres retractor is replaced superotemporally. Then, the Bishop tendon tucker is repositioned through the tucked portion of the tendon, and the polyester suture is released and removed.

d) The tendon tucker is then adjusted for a larger or smaller tuck, and the polyester suture is replaced at the base of the tucked tendon as previously described.

12. Once the appropriate tucking of the superior oblique tendon is confirmed, the bowtie slipknot in the polyester suture is converted to a permanent knot with an additional 1-throw knot for a 3–1-1 throw square knot. One end of the trimmed suture can be passed through the tucked tendon to tack down the "knee" of the tendon to sclera temporally with a partial-thickness scleral pass. The needles are then trimmed.

13. All instruments are removed, and the conjunctival incision is reapproximated and usually does not require sutured closure.

7.8.5 Harada-Ito Procedure[5]

The Harada-Ito procedure is often performed bilaterally. Alternative techniques for tightening the anterior fibers of the superior oblique tendon have been described. For the Fells modification, the anterior fibers are disinserted and then reinserted 7 to 8 mm posterior to the superior pole of the lateral rectus insertion.[4] Another technique is tucking of the anterior fibers of the superior oblique tendon,[6] which eliminates the need for a scleral pass laterally:

1. Indirect ophthalmoscopy after pupillary dilation is first performed to evaluate fundus extorsion.

2. A fornix incision is made in the superotemporal quadrant using blunt Westcott scissors, approximately 8 mm posterior to the limbus.

3. The superior rectus muscle is isolated first with a Stevens hook, and then with a Jameson hook, which is swept toward the limbus to ensure that the entire width of the muscle has been isolated.

4. A Stevens hook is used to reflect the conjunctiva over the bulb of the Jameson hook.

5. Blunt Westcott scissors are used to make an incision in the intermuscular septum just under the bulb of the Jameson hook, and a Stevens hook is inserted in the opening to perform a pole test to confirm that the entire width of the superior rectus muscle has been isolated.

6. A small Desmarres retractor is then placed in the conjunctival incision to expose the temporal aspect of the superior rectus muscle. The Jameson hook is used to displace the superior rectus nasally.

7. A Stevens hook, with its tip pointed nasally, is swept posteriorly along the temporal border of the superior rectus muscle to the posterior margin of the white fibers of the superior oblique tendon, which is isolated onto the hook, with care to hook the entire tendon but avoiding the superotemporal vortex vein. The anterior half of the distal tendon is carefully cleared of connective tissue with blunt dissection.

8. The anterior one-third of the superior oblique tendon is then isolated onto a second Stevens hook and split from the posterior two-thirds of the tendon as far nasally as possible with the second Stevens hook.

9. The separated anterior tendon near or just under the temporal aspect of the superior rectus muscle is secured with a 6–0 double-armed polyglactin suture with partial-thickness passes of each needle across the width of the anterior tendon in opposite directions, followed by full-thickness locking bites at either edge of the separated anterior tendon. The Jameson hook on the superior rectus muscle is then removed.

10. The lateral rectus muscle is isolated onto a Stevens hook, followed by a Jameson hook. The Stevens hook is then used to retract the conjunctiva to expose the superior aspect of the lateral rectus insertion and muscle.

11. Using calipers, 7 to 8 mm posterior to the superior pole of the lateral rectus insertion is marked. The anterior tendon suture is inserted at the marked location with partial-thickness scleral passes. The eye can be rotated superonasally using the Jameson hook on the lateral rectus muscle, as the suture is pulled through the scleral tunnels, for the tendon to reach the superior aspect of the lateral rectus muscle as far as possible. The tendon suture is then tied with a 3–1 throw bowtie slipknot.

12. Steps 2 to 11 are repeated for the superior oblique tendon in the fellow eye.
13. Indirect ophthalmoscopy is repeated to evaluate fundus torsion, with the goal of no torsion to slight intorsion in both eyes. If the tendon has been positioned to be as close as possible to the lateral rectus, there may be limited capacity to tighten further, but the tendon can be allowed to hang back if the eyes are excessively intorted.
14. Once bilateral fundus torsion is satisfactory, the bowtie slipknots in both eyes are converted to permanent knots with an additional 1-throw knot for a 3–1–1 throw square knot. The suture is then trimmed.
15. All instruments are removed, and the conjunctival incision is reapproximated and usually does not require sutured closure.

7.9 Tips and Pearls

- Surrounding fascia can initially obscure visualization of the superior oblique tendon which appears as glistening fibers running nearly perpendicular to the superior rectus muscle and flush against the globe.
- The authors prefer intraoperative adjustment for superior oblique surgery over postoperative adjustment, which can be challenging and more uncomfortable for the patient compared to adjustable rectus muscle surgery.
- A headlight is helpful but not required to visualize the more posteriorly located superior oblique tendon.

7.9.1 Superior Oblique Weakening Procedures

- Superior oblique surgery for congenital or acquired Brown syndrome is reserved for those patients with significant ocular torticollis due to a vertical deviation in primary gaze. Some congenital cases have been reported to resolve with age,[7]and some acquired cases may resolve with local or systemic steroid treatment.
- Either a superotemporal or a superonasal conjunctival incision may be used to access the nasal superior oblique tendon, the latter being used to better preserve the nasal intermuscular septum.
- Superior oblique weakening procedures are performed nasal to the superior rectus muscle where the tendon is narrower and more easily

completely hooked to decrease the risk of undercorrection.
- Superior oblique tenotomy is considered more potent if performed closer to the trochlea.
- When placing the superior oblique suture spacer, some surgeons first secure the nonabsorbable suture at the nasal aspect of the tendon, and then pass the suture through the temporal aspect of the tendon, adjacent to the superior rectus muscle due to concern for iatrogenic Brown syndrome if the adjustable ends of the suture are positioned nasally, possibly resulting in scarring at the trochlea. However, temporally positioned ends of the adjustable suture may be more difficult to access and adjust if they are under the superior rectus muscle.
- Superior oblique Z-tenotomy,[8] split tendon elongation,[9] and the silicone band spacer,[10] not included in this chapter, are alternative techniques to lengthen the superior oblique tendon. Recession of the superior oblique tendon is not recommended due to the far posterior reattachment of the posterior fibers required to avoid anti-depression.

7.9.2 Superior Oblique Tightening Procedures

- The approach to unilateral trochlear nerve paresis is surgeon-dependent. Some surgeons weaken the ipsilateral inferior oblique muscle, as described in Chapter 6, as first-line surgical treatment. Other surgeons tighten the affected superior oblique tendon as first-line surgical treatment.
- When hooking the distal superior oblique tendon which fans out posteriorly at its insertion, care is taken to avoid injuring the superotemporal vortex vein, usually located at the junction between the anterior two-thirds and posterior one-third of the superior oblique tendon, near the temporal aspect of the superior rectus muscle.
- Unmasking of a bilateral superior oblique paresis can occur when unilateral surgery is performed due to marked asymmetry of the measurements, resulting in the preoperative appearance of a unilateral abnormality. Bilateral superior oblique paresis is suspected in patients who have more than 10 to 12 degrees of extorsion on double Maddox rod testing, alternating hypertropia, large esotropia in downgaze often resulting in a chin down head position, and bilateral fundus extorsion.

- For superior oblique tucks, when evaluating the tightness of the superior oblique tendon by adducting and elevating the globe, ensure that the eye is neither proptosed nor retropulsed, which will result in an inaccurate assessment of Saunder's forced duction testing.
- In patients with torsional diplopia, improvement of torsion to less than 4 to 6 degrees following the Harada-Ito procedure improves the patient's ability to fuse postoperatively,[11] as torsional fusional amplitudes are typically 6 to 8 degrees.

7.10 What to Avoid

- Avoid blind hooking of the superior oblique tendon.
- Avoid suture placement and handling of the superior oblique tendon too far nasally near the trochlea, which can result in iatrogenic Brown syndrome due to scarring.
- Careful dissection of the fascia surrounding the superior oblique tendon helps minimize scar formation and maintain the anatomic relationships of the tendon.

7.11 Complications

- Injury to the overlying superior rectus muscle.
- Injury to the superotemporal vortex vein.
- Orbital fat adherence due to violation of Tenon's capsule posteriorly if dissection of Tenon's capsule and hooking of the tendon is attempted without adequate visualization.
- Overcorrection of deviation:
  - Iatrogenic Brown syndrome due to excess tucking of the superior oblique tendon or scarring near the trochlea.
  - Excess weakening of the superior oblique tendon resulting in the appearance of a superior oblique paresis, particularly after surgery for Brown syndrome, for which the goal of surgery is a small undercorrection.
- Undercorrection of the deviation:
  - Incomplete transection of the tendon due to residual intact tendon fibers following superior oblique tenotomy, which can be detected with repeat exaggerated traction testing.

7.12 Postoperative Care

- Surgical treatment of torsional diplopia may require a longer period of adjustment in the postoperative period.
- Following superior oblique surgery, patients with significant astigmatism should be refracted postoperatively to account for the change in the astigmatism axis.[9]

References

[1] Helveston EM, Giangiacomo JG, Ellis FD. Congenital absence of the superior oblique tendon. Trans Am Ophthalmol Soc. 1981; 79:123–135

[2] von Noorden GK, Olivier P. Superior oblique tenectomy in Brown's syndrome. Ophthalmology. 1982; 89(4):303–309

[3] Guyton DL. Exaggerated traction test for the oblique muscles. Ophthalmology. 1981; 88(10):1035–1040

[4] Del Monte MA, Archer SM. Atlas of Pediatric Ophthalmology and Strabismus. New York, NY: Churchill Livingstone; 1993

[5] Harada M, Ito Y. Visual correction of cyclotropia. Jpn J Ophthalmol. 1964; 8:88–96

[6] Pineles SL, Velez FG. Anterior superior oblique tuck: an alternate treatment for excyclotorsion. J AAPOS. 2018; 22(5):393–393.e1

[7] Lambert SR. Late spontaneous resolution of congenital Brown syndrome. J AAPOS. 2010; 14(4):373–375

[8] Brooks DR, Morrison DG, Donahue SP. The efficacy of superior oblique Z-tenotomy in the treatment of overdepression in adduction (superior oblique overaction). J AAPOS. 2012; 16(4):342–344

[9] Kushner BJ. Strabismus: practical pearls you won't find in textbooks. Cham, Switzerland: Springer; 2017

[10] Wright KW. Color atlas of strabismus surgery: strategies and techniques, 3rd ed. New York, NY: Springer; 2007

[11] Georgievski Z, Sleep M, Koklanis K. Simulated torsional disparity disrupts horizontal fusion and stereopsis. J AAPOS. 2007; 11(2):120–124

8 Reoperations

Sylvia H. Yoo

Summary

Reoperations in strabismus surgery can pose a challenge for the surgeon, as the surgery is typically less predictable and scar tissue may be present. Prior operative reports are also not always available, although clues during the preoperative history and examination, such as the patient family's recall of the original deviation and evidence of conjunctival scarring, as well as exploration of the muscles during surgery are useful in finalizing the surgical plan. This chapter focuses on reoperation of the rectus muscles, but the principles can be applied to the oblique muscles as well.

Keywords: reoperation, recurrent strabismus, residual strabismus, overcorrection, stretch scar

8.1 Goals

The goal of a reoperation in strabismus surgery is to improve a recurrent or residual strabismus, or correct an overcorrection of prior surgery while preserving the blood supply of the anterior segment, minimizing additional scar formation, and aiming for an optimal long-term surgical outcome with the hopes of not needing additional surgery. Minimizing additional scar formation decreases the risk of restriction, may improve cosmesis and patient discomfort, and lessens the difficulty of future reoperations if they are needed.

8.2 Advantages

In most cases, strabismus surgery on an extraocular muscle can be performed multiple times, keeping in mind that with each surgery, additional scar tissue can develop, further altering normal surgical anatomy and increasing the difficulty of subsequent surgery.

8.3 Expectations

The rate of reoperation in strabismus surgery in the United States has been reported to be 6.7% within one year after strabismus surgery.[1] This rate may be higher beyond the first year after surgery. The expectation of additional strabismus surgery is improvement of persistent strabismus, which may or may not be associated with diplopia.[1]

8.4 Key Principles

- Prior operative reports, if available, are reviewed to determine the original deviation, the muscles that were operated on, and the amount of surgery that was performed.
- Assessment of conjunctival scarring, versions and ductions, the presence of secondary deviations, as well as intraoperative forced duction testing are used for surgical planning for reoperations.
- Anticipate and address the presence of scar tissue if additional surgery is being performed on previously operated muscle(s). A fornix incision may be used in reoperations and is described in this chapter, but some surgeons prefer limbal incisions for greater exposure. In some cases, exploration of the extraocular muscles is needed to determine or confirm the sites of insertion, and to determine the final surgical plan.
- Reoperations of rectus muscles include re-recession or advancement of previously recessed muscles and re-resection or recession of previously resected muscles.

8.5 Indications

Recurrent strabismus and overcorrections, which can occur months to years following prior strabismus surgery.

8.6 Contraindications

For patients who have previously undergone multiple eye muscle surgeries on multiple extraocular muscles for complex strabismus, the potential benefits and risks of additional surgery should be understood by the family. If the expectations are not realistic or the expected benefits are deemed to be potentially outweighed by the risks, additional surgery may not be recommended but can be considered again at a later time if the deviation persists or changes.

8.7 Preoperative Preparation

If the patient has a history of strabismus surgery done elsewhere, obtain as much history as possible from the patient and from the patient's medical records, which may require contacting the patient's former surgeon or the hospital where the surgery was performed. Examine the patient for evidence of prior surgery, such as conjunctival scarring and limited ductions. Intraoperative forced duction testing is essential for final surgical planning. Prepare the patient and family for postoperative discomfort, which may be more significant if scar tissue is encountered and dissected, and for the possibility of needing additional surgery in the future.

8.8 Operative Technique

1. Forced duction testing is performed as described in Chapter 4.8.1 Forced Duction Testing to provide additional information for final surgical planning.
2. Once the operative rectus muscle has been isolated onto a Jameson or Guyton hook, the bulb of the hook is swept toward the limbus to aid in determining if the entire width of the muscle has been hooked and also whether there is significant subconjunctival scarring.
3. If subconjunctival scarring is suspected, careful blunt dissection is performed with blunt Westcott scissors between the conjunctiva and the muscle, including the space across the width of the muscle and posteriorly (▶ Fig. 8.1). The space between the conjunctiva and sclera

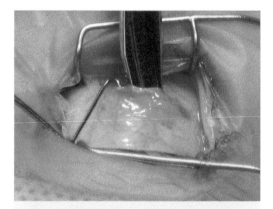

Fig. 8.1 If subconjunctival scarring is present, blunt dissection is performed between the conjunctiva and the muscle after it is hooked.

anterior to the insertion is also bluntly dissected. Sharp dissection may be needed for robust scar tissue, which should be first visualized as much as possible, and is performed with care to avoid cutting the muscle or vessels.
4. Once the scar tissue seems to be adequately released, the closed blades of the Westcott scissors should be able to glide relatively smoothly over the muscle from anterior to its insertion toward the muscle belly, and across the width of the muscle. The conjunctiva is then carefully draped over the bulb of the muscle hook with a Stevens hook.
5. The surgery then proceeds with the steps described in Chapter 4 for weakening or tightening of the operative muscles, keeping in mind that additional scar tissue may be encountered:
    a) Scar tissue includes formation of stretch scar between the insertion site and the muscle, which effectively weakens the muscle. Stretch scar may appear striated, similar to muscle, but can be differentiated with close inspection and mindfulness of normal anatomy. Stretch scar is typically resected if present.

8.9 Tips and Pearls

- Even when operating on previously untouched muscles, the prior surgery may affect the outcome. For example, a rectus muscle resection may be more potent in the setting of a previously recessed antagonist muscle.
- While it may be preferable to operate on an untouched muscle to avoid scar tissue, surgery on previously operated muscles is indicated in some cases. For example, a patient with an exotropia following medial rectus recession for a history of esotropia may undergo lateral rectus recession, but if adduction is limited or if the exotropia at near is larger than at distance, advancement of the previously recessed medial rectus muscles is indicated.
- Intraoperative forced duction testing is useful not only prior to the start of surgery but may also be repeated during surgery to confirm adequate release of restrictive scar tissue.
- In some cases, dissection and release of exuberant scarring and adhesions around the extraocular muscles may be adequate to resolve restriction causing the strabismus.
- Surgery on a previously operated muscle is less predictable and the use of adjustable sutures may be warranted in appropriate settings.[2]

– Small re-recession of a previously recessed muscle may result in a relatively large effect.
– Advancement of a previously recessed muscle may result in a relatively small effect; thus, a small resection may be included with the advancement.
– Recession of a previously resected muscle may be more potent than recession of an unoperated muscle.
– Re-resection of a previously resected muscle may have slightly greater effect than resection of an unoperated muscle.
• In patients with a history of multiple reoperations and significant scarring, subconjunctival dexamethasone may be considered to lessen additional scar formation.

8.10 What to Avoid

• Inadvertently cutting the muscle or vessels during dissection and release of scar tissue.
• Misidentification of stretch scar as muscle.
• Excess manipulation of tissue which may lead to greater scar formation.

8.11 Complications

• Significant scar formation causing restriction, discomfort, poor cosmesis, and possibly complicating future surgeries if needed.
• Anterior segment ischemia.
• The patient should be aware of the risks of undercorrection and overcorrection even after additional surgery.

8.12 Postoperative Care

• If significant scarring is dissected intraoperatively, a longer course of postoperative topical corticosteroid may be considered with monitoring of the intraocular pressure.

References

[1] Repka MX, Lum F, Burugapalli B. Strabismus, strabismus surgery, and reoperation rate in the United States: analysis from the IRIS registry. Ophthalmology. 2018; 125(10):1646–1653
[2] Del Monte MA, Archer SM. Atlas of pediatric ophthalmology and strabismus surgery. New York, NY: Churchill Livingstone; 1993

9 Special Strabismus Procedures

Catherine S. Choi and Sylvia H. Yoo

Summary

A variety of strabismus surgery techniques have been described to address complex types of strabismus. This chapter describes a number of these strabismus procedures, most of which alter the vector forces of the operative muscles with or without concomitant tightening or weakening procedures. These procedures may be kept in the surgeon's armamentarium to improve the eye alignment in patients with complex strabismus. Bear in mind that this chapter is not all-inclusive of the innovative strabismus surgery techniques that have been described, and additional techniques are mentioned with references for further study.

Keywords: complex strabismus, transposition, posterior fixation, Y-split procedure, partial tendon recession, cranial nerve palsy, Duane syndrome, upshoot, downshoot, diplopia

9.1 Goals

In addition to the goals of all strabismus surgery described in Chapter 1.1 Goals, the specific goals of the procedures described in this chapter.

9.1.1 Transposition Procedures

Improve eye alignment in patients with poor function of a rectus muscle by tethering the eye in the direction of the weak muscle's field of action.

9.1.2 Posterior Fixation Sutures

Weaken a rectus muscle in its field of action, by creating an ancillary insertion posterior to the insertion, without overcorrecting the alignment in other gaze positions. Innervation to the yoke muscle is, in turn, increased which may also serve as a mechanism to improve the alignment.

9.1.3 Y-split Procedure of the Lateral Rectus Muscle

Improve an isolated upshoot or downshoot in Duane syndrome caused by co-contraction (leash phenomenon) of the horizontal rectus muscles in adduction by broadening the lateral rectus insertion to stabilize the position of the lateral rectus muscle and prevent it from shifting superiorly or inferiorly over the globe. If significant globe retraction and associated enophthalmos are present, large recessions (approximately 10 mm) of both the medial and lateral rectus muscles can also correct an upshoot or downshoot, without the need for the Y-split procedure.

9.1.4 Partial Tendon Recession

Resolve diplopia secondary to small-angle vertical deviations, eliminating the need for prism glasses.

9.2 Advantages

- Familiarity with these procedures allows the surgeon to offer additional surgical options to patients when discussing the optimal approach for complex types of strabismus.
- A transposition procedure is more effective than a recess-resect procedure for a complete abducens nerve palsy, which is not recommended, as resection of a completely paretic lateral rectus muscle is unlikely to result in long-term improvement of alignment and precludes transposition of the vertical rectus muscles due to risk of anterior segment ischemia.

9.3 Expectations

- Improvement of eye alignment is the primary expectation for strabismus surgery.
- Following transposition and Y-split procedures, the expectation should *not* be for normalization of ocular motility.
- Incomitance of strabismus is expected to improve with posterior fixation, and elimination of the need for prism glasses is expected after the partial tendon procedure.

9.4 Key Principles

- These procedures may be used with concomitant muscle weakening or tightening procedures if indicated, keeping in mind any prior strabismus surgeries and the risk of anterior segment ischemia if multiple rectus muscles are disinserted.

- Some of the procedures described require far posterior exposure to effectively alter the force vectors of the muscles.

9.5 Indications

9.5.1 Transposition Procedures

Any condition in which a rectus muscle has poor function, usually due to abnormal innervation, which may be congenital or acquired.
- Abducens nerve (6th cranial nerve) paresis with little to no function of the lateral rectus muscle, resulting in an esotropia.
- Duane syndrome, particularly esotropic Duane syndrome with poor abduction.
- Monocular elevation deficiency without restriction of the inferior rectus muscle.
- Slipped rectus muscle that is iatrogenic or due to trauma, if it is unable to be recovered or with persistent underaction of the muscle.
- Oculomotor nerve (3rd cranial nerve) paresis
  - Exotropia and hypotropia are usually present, but the deviation is dependent on the degree of involvement of the superior and inferior divisions of the oculomotor nerve which dictates the surgical management.
  - Medial transposition of the lateral rectus,[1] passed between the sclera and both the vertical rectus and obliques muscles with the aid of a Gass hook to reach the medial rectus insertion, has been described.
  - Maximal but reversible weakening of the lateral rectus muscle by fixation with nonabsorbable suture to the periosteum of the orbital wall[2] may also be considered.
- Rare cases of congenitally absent rectus muscle(s).

9.5.2 Posterior Fixation Sutures

- Esotropia with convergence excess (high AC/A).
- Incomitant strabismus by operating on the yoke muscle on the unaffected fellow eye to balance it with the underacting muscle in the affected eye. For example, for a left abducens nerve paresis with a large secondary deviation of the right medial rectus muscle in left gaze but with a smaller esotropia in primary gaze, a posterior fixation suture may be placed on the right medial rectus muscle in addition to horizontal rectus muscle surgery in the left eye.

9.5.3 Y-split Procedure of the Lateral Rectus Muscle

The Y-split procedure of the lateral rectus muscle is performed specifically for Duane syndrome with an upshoot or downshoot.

9.5.4 Partial Tendon Recession

Symptomatic diplopia from small-angle vertical strabismus and desire for independence from prism glasses, such as a patient with diplopia who would like to play sports without the need for prism glasses.

9.6 Contraindications

In addition to the contraindications of all strabismus surgeries described in Chapter 1.6 Contraindications, disinsertion of multiple rectus muscles increases the risk of anterior segment ischemia, including in rare cases of congenitally absent rectus muscles.

9.7 Preoperative Preparation

A complete sensorimotor examination is performed as described in Chapter 1.7 Preoperative Preparation. In addition, any prior operative reports are reviewed, if available. Though rare, if there is suspicion for congenital absence of rectus muscles, imaging is warranted.[3] Intraoperative forced duction testing is also important for final surgical planning. Ensure that patients with abnormal innervation of the extraocular muscles understand that the motility will not be normalized with strabismus surgery.

9.8 Operative Technique

9.8.1 Transposition Procedures

For a weak lateral rectus muscle, the superior rectus or both vertical rectus muscles are transposed and inserted adjacent to the lateral rectus insertion. For monocular elevation deficiency without significant tightness of the inferior rectus, a similar technique is used for superior transposition of the medial and lateral rectus muscles (Knapp procedure).

Several transposition techniques have been described:
- Full tendon transposition is described below.
- The Hummelsheim procedure, which is a partial tendon transposition of the vertical rectus muscles, spares the anterior ciliary vessels at the

nondisinserted halves of the transposed rectus muscles.

- The Jensen procedure also splits the transposed muscles but without disinsertion, joining the adjacent half of the transposed muscle to the weak muscle with a nonabsorbable polyester suture. While it is theoretically a vessel sparing procedure, anterior segment ischemia has been reported.[4] It is technically difficult and may result in greater scarring than the other techniques, making reoperations more challenging.

A fornix incision is created in the quadrant between the weak muscle and the muscle to be transposed. If two muscles are transposed, two fornix incisions are used. For example, superotemporal and inferotemporal fornix incisions are used for transpositions of the vertical rectus muscles to a weak lateral rectus muscle:

1. The rectus muscle to be transposed is isolated on a muscle hook and cleared of its overlying Tenon's capsule and connective tissue with blunt dissection, which should be performed far posteriorly for transposition of vertical rectus muscles to avoid significant changes in the upper and lower eyelid positions. The fascial connection between the superior rectus and the superior oblique tendon should also be separated to decrease the risk of an unexpected vertical deviation.
2. The muscle is secured on a 6–0 double-armed polyglactin suture near its insertion and disinserted as described in Chapter 4.8.3 Rectus Muscle Recession.
3. The weak muscle is then isolated on a Jameson or Guyton muscle hook through the same fornix incision, clearing with blunt dissection the corresponding pole of the muscle to bare sclera where the transposed muscle will be reattached.
4. The disinserted muscle is then reattached adjacent to the weak muscle (▶ Fig. 9.1). The pole of the transposed muscle proximal to the weak muscle can be reinserted just posterior to the corresponding pole of the weak muscle, while the distal pole of the transposed muscle is reinserted adjacent to the weak muscle, so that the center of the insertion of the transposed muscle is at the pole of the weak muscle.

Modifications of transposition to augment its effect include:

- Scleral fixation using 6–0 nonabsorbable polyester suture of approximately one-fourth of the width of the transposed muscle belly to the

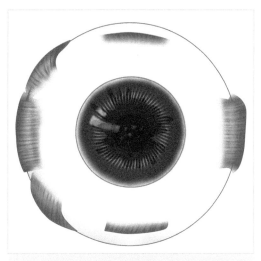

Fig. 9.1 The superior and inferior rectus muscles have been transposed to the weak lateral rectus muscle.

sclera, adjacent to the weak muscle. This is performed far posteriorly at least 12 to 14 mm posterior to the insertion of the weak muscle and may be technically difficult.

- Union of approximately one-fourth of the width of the transposed muscle belly to the adjacent one-fourth width of the weak muscle with a 6–0 nonabsorbable polyester suture, 5 to 6 mm posterior to the insertion of the weak muscle.[5]

9.8.2 Posterior Fixation Sutures

Either a fornix incision or a limbal incision may be used, although a limbal incision allows better posterior exposure of the sclera. Posterior fixation is usually performed with concomitant recession of the muscle, allowing the posterior sclera to be more readily exposed while the muscle is disinserted:

1. The rectus muscle is secured on a 6–0 double-armed polyglactin suture near its insertion and disinserted as described in Chapter 4.8.3 Rectus Muscle Recession.
2. Using calipers or a curved Scott ruler, 12 to 14 mm posterior to the center of the original insertion is measured and marked on bare sclera. A double-armed 6–0 nonabsorbable polyester suture is placed at the marked location with a partial-thickness scleral pass that is parallel to the insertion.[5] A secure grasp with toothed forceps at the original insertion is required to maintain adequate exposure and stable rotation of the globe during the posteriorly located scleral pass.

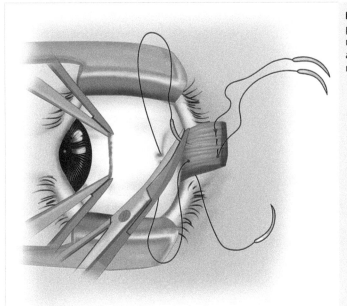

Fig. 9.2 The partial-thickness scleral pass for a posterior fixation suture is made while the muscle is disinserted if a concomitant recession of the rectus muscle is planned.

3. The needles on the nonabsorbable suture are then moved away from the center of the surgical field.
4. The muscle is then reinserted at the planned recessed insertion site.
5. Each needle on the preplaced nonabsorbable suture is then passed from under the muscle belly toward its surface 12 to 14 mm from the original insertion and approximately one-third of the width from each the edge of the muscle. A Stevens hook can be used to elevate the edge of the muscle:
   a) Alternatively, before the muscle is disinserted, the location of the muscle belly that will lie 12 to 14 mm posterior to the original insertion following the planned recession is identified. Here, a 6–0 double-armed nonabsorbable suture is placed approximately one-third of the width from one edge of the muscle, by passing the needle from under the muscle to its surface.[6] A Stevens hook can be used to elevate the edge of the muscle. The muscle is then disinserted. Using calipers or a curved Scott ruler, 12 to 14 mm posterior to the center of the original insertion is measured and marked on the sclera. The needle on the nonabsorbable suture from under the muscle belly is used to place a partial-thickness scleral pass parallel to the insertion at the marked location. A secure grasp with toothed forceps at the original insertion is required to maintain adequate exposure and stable rotation

of the globe during the posteriorly located scleral pass. The same needle is then passed approximately one-third of the width from the other edge of the muscle, directly across from the first pass (▶ Fig. 9.2). The muscle is then reinserted at the planned recessed insertion site.
6. Ensuring that any hidden slack is taken out of the nonabsorbable suture, the ends of the suture are securely tied with a 1–1 throw square knot over the muscle belly without overtightening the knot, which can result in muscle necrosis.

If a rectus muscle recession is not planned at the time of posterior fixation suture placement, the procedure is performed with two separate single-armed nonabsorbable sutures (or double-armed suture cut in half):
1. The operative muscle is isolated on a muscle hook to maximally rotate the eye away from its field of action. Overlying connective tissue is bluntly dissected far posteriorly to expose the muscle belly.
2. Calipers or a curved Scott ruler is used to measure and mark 12 to 14 mm posterior to the insertion on sclera.
3. A Stevens hook elevates one edge of the muscle, and a 6–0 nonabsorbable polyester suture is placed at the marked location with a partial-thickness scleral pass just under the edge of the muscle.

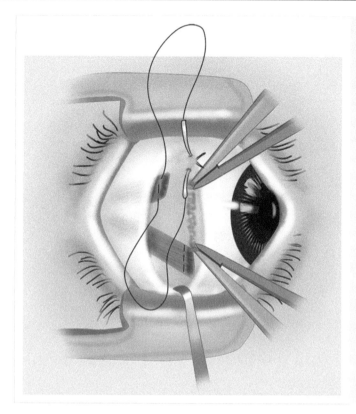

Fig. 9.3 For the Y-split procedure, the superior and inferior halves of the lateral rectus muscle are reattached with the inferior border of the superior half at the superior pole of the original insertion and the superior border of the inferior half at the inferior pole of the insertion.

4. The Stevens hook is then removed, and the needle is passed from under the muscle toward its surface to include approximately one-fourth of the width of the muscle. The suture is tied down to secure the posterior muscle belly at this position.
5. The procedure is repeated at the opposite edge of the muscle, 12 to 14 mm posterior to the insertion.

9.8.3 Y-split Procedure of the Lateral Rectus Muscle

1. The lateral rectus is isolated through an inferotemporal fornix incision, and the overlying Tenon's capsule and connective tissue are cleared from the muscle far posteriorly.
2. The muscle is bluntly split into equal halves from its insertion to 14 to 15 mm posterior to the insertion using two Stevens hooks. Westcott scissors are used if needed.
3. Two separate double-armed 6–0 polyglactin sutures are used to secure each half of the muscle at the insertion with partial-thickness passes to either edge of the muscle half and full-thickness locking bites.

4. Each half of the muscle is disinserted using blunt Westcott scissors.
5. The two halves of the lateral rectus muscle are reattached with partial-thickness scleral passes as follows: the inferior border of the superior half is reattached at the superior pole of the original insertion, and the superior border of the inferior half is reattached at the inferior pole of the insertion (▶ Fig. 9.3).

9.8.4 Partial Tendon Recession

For a partial tendon procedure, the amount of recession is 1.0 mm for every 1.5 prism diopters of vertical deviation.[7]

1. An eyelid speculum is placed in the operative eye, and a fornix incision is made parallel to the eyelid margin using blunt Westcott scissors (superotemporal or superonasal quadrant for superior rectus surgery and inferotemporal or inferonasal quadrant for inferior rectus surgery), approximately 8 mm posterior to the limbus.
2. The vertical rectus muscle is isolated with a Stevens hook, followed by a Jameson hook, which is swept toward the limbus to ensure

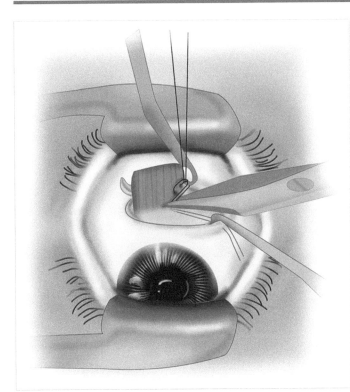

Fig. 9.4 For the partial tendon procedure, imbricate and disinsert one pole of the vertical muscle, sparing one anterior ciliary vessel.

that the entire width of the muscle has been isolated.

3. A Stevens hook is used to reflect the conjunctiva over the bulb of the Jameson hook.

4. Westcott scissors are used to incise the intermuscular septum overlying the bulb of the Jameson hook, and a Stevens hook is inserted in the opening to perform a pole test, ensuring that the entire vertical rectus muscle has been isolated.

5. Anterior and posterior connective tissue overlying the muscle and its insertion is bluntly and sharply dissected with Westcott scissors.

6. A 6–0 single-armed polyglactin suture is used to secure one pole of the tendon by first passing the suture partial thickness from the outer edge of the tendon toward the center, followed by a full-thickness pass of approximately one-fourth of the width of the tendon. The suture is locked by passing the needle through the suture loop.

7. The imbricated pole of the tendon is disinserted to within 2 mm of the opposite pole, so that approximately seven-eighths of the width of the tendon is disinserted. The anterior ciliary vessel at the opposite pole is visualized and should remain intact (▶ Fig. 9.4).

8. The disinserted pole is reattached to the sclera by the planned amount of recession.

9. The pole suture is secured with a 3–1–1 throw square knot at this position, resulting in a diagonal line from the intact pole of the tendon to the recessed pole (▶ Fig. 9.5).

10. The overlying conjunctiva is massaged to reapproximate the wound, usually not requiring sutured closure.

9.9 Tips and Pearls

9.9.1 Transposition Procedures

- The decision for the transposition technique to be used is dependent on the surgeon's preference and the patient's risk of anterior segment ischemia. Recall that fornix incisions may better preserve the anterior segment circulation.
- If a split tendon procedure is performed, principles similar to the full tendon transposition technique are used:
  - Only the overlying connective tissue on the side of the muscle to be transposed is bluntly dissected.
  - The muscle is split as far posteriorly as possible, approximately 12 to 15 mm posterior to the insertion.

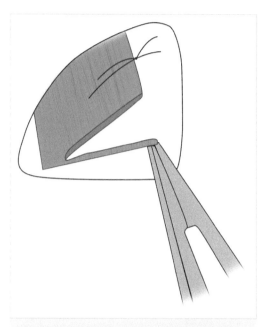

Fig. 9.5 For the partial tendon procedure, recess the pole of the vertical muscle by the planned amount based on the preoperative deviation.

- A weakening procedure of the antagonist rectus muscle of the weak muscle, either with rectus muscle recession or with botulinum toxin, is usually performed in conjunction with a transposition procedure, keeping in mind the number of rectus muscles that are disinserted.
- For abducens nerve palsy or esotropic Duane syndrome, transposition of only the superior rectus muscle has been described with successful postoperative outcomes and without development of torsional or vertical diplopia.[8] The risk of anterior segment ischemia is also decreased. The fascial connection between the superior rectus and the superior oblique tendon should be separated to decrease the risk of an unexpected vertical deviation.

9.9.2 Posterior Fixation Sutures

- A short, spatulated needle should be used for placement of the posterior scleral passes.
- Posterior fixation sutures must be placed as far posteriorly as possible, at least 12 to 14 mm posterior to the original insertion, to be effective.

- Posterior fixation suture placement is challenging due to the far posterior exposure required, putting the globe at greater risk of scleral perforation during placement of the partial-thickness scleral pass and is only used in select cases. A malleable ribbon retractor can be helpful in providing the posterior exposure needed.

9.9.3 Y-split Procedure of the Lateral Rectus Muscle

- Maintain the width of each half of the muscle when reinserting the split muscle.
- For esotropic Duane syndrome with an esotropia in primary gaze or head turn, medial rectus recession can be performed at the time of the Y-split procedure on the lateral rectus muscle.
- For exotropic Duane syndrome, the split lateral rectus halves can also be recessed, measured from the superior and inferior poles of the original insertion.[9]
- The distance between the reinserted halves of the muscle should be at least the width of the original insertion to treat the upshoot or downshoot effectively.
- Without a recession of the lateral rectus muscle, the Y-split procedure should not affect the horizontal alignment.

9.9.4 Partial Tendon Recession

- A 1.0 mm full tendon recession of a vertical rectus muscle treats approximately 3 prism diopters of vertical strabismus; thus, a 1.0 mm partial tendon recession of a vertical rectus muscle corrects approximately 1.5 prism diopters of vertical strabismus. Generally, the maximum amount of recession is 5.0 mm for the partial tendon recession.
- The pole to be recessed can be selected to help correct preoperative torsion, if present. To correct preoperative intorsion, the temporal pole of the superior rectus or the nasal pole of the inferior rectus muscle is recessed. Likewise, for preoperative extorsion, the nasal pole of the superior rectus or temporal pole of the inferior rectus is recessed.
- The decision to operate on the superior rectus of one eye versus the inferior rectus of the fellow eye depends on whether the vertical deviation is greater in the upgaze or downgaze position. If no incomitance is present, either the superior rectus or the inferior rectus may be

chosen, keeping in mind that the partial tendon procedure on the superior rectus may have a higher risk of undercorrection,[7] while the inferior rectus may have a higher risk of overcorrection and is more likely to affect downgaze and reading positions.

9.10 What to Avoid

- Disinsertion of three or more rectus muscles if a transposition procedure is planned.
- Asymmetric muscle reinsertion during transposition if two rectus muscles are transposed, which may result in new vertical and/or torsional deviations.
- Scleral perforation during placement of posterior fixation sutures, possibly due to inadequate posterior exposure.

9.11 Complications

In addition to the risks described in Chapter 1.11 Complications:

- Development of torsion and/or vertical deviation in transposition procedures and theoretically, torsional diplopia in partial tendon procedures.
- Ineffectiveness of posterior fixation suture placement despite far posterior scleral passes.
- Anterior segment ischemia is a risk, especially with disinsertion of three or more rectus muscles in transposition procedures. Alternative techniques may need to be considered.

- Procedures requiring far posterior partial-thickness scleral passes increase the risk of scleral perforation.

9.12 Postoperative Care

See Chapter 1.12, Postoperative Care.

References

[1] Gokyigit B, Akar S, Satana B, Demirok A, Yilmaz OF. Medial transposition of a split lateral rectus muscle for complete oculomotor nerve palsy. J AAPOS. 2013; 17(4):402–410

[2] Velez FG, Thacker N, Britt MT, Alcorn D, Foster RS, Rosenbaum AL. Rectus muscle orbital wall fixation: a reversible profound weakening procedure. J AAPOS. 2004; 8(5):473–480

[3] Astle WF, Hill VE, Ells AL, Chi NT, Martinovic E. Congenital absence of the inferior rectus muscle: diagnosis and management. J AAPOS. 2003; 7(5):339–344

[4] Bleik JH, Cherfan GM. Anterior segment ischemia after the Jensen procedure in a 10-year-old patient. Am J Ophthalmol. 1995; 119(4):524–525

[5] Wright KW. Color Atlas of strabismus surgery: strategies and techniques, 3rd ed. New York, NY: Springer; 2007

[6] Del Monte MA, Archer SM. Atlas of pediatric ophthalmology and strabismus surgery. New York, NY: Churchill Livingstone; 1993

[7] Singh J, Choi CS, Bahl R, Archer SM. Partial tendon recession for small-angle vertical strabismus. J AAPOS. 2016; 20(5): 392–395

[8] Mehendale RA, Dagi LR, Wu C, Ledoux D, Johnston S, Hunter DG. Superior rectus transposition and medial rectus recession for Duane syndrome and sixth nerve palsy. Arch Ophthalmol. 2012; 130(2):195–201

[9] Velez FG, Velez G, Hendler K, Pineles SL. Isolated Y-splitting and recession of the lateral rectus muscle in patients with exo-Duane syndrome. Strabismus. 2012; 20(3):109–114

10 Botulinum Toxin Injection for Strabismus

Sylvia H. Yoo

Summary

Botulinum toxin can be used as an alternate muscle weakening procedure in place of incisional surgery or as an adjunct to incisional surgery.

Keywords: botulinum toxin, onabotulinum toxin A, esotropia, chemodenervation, ptosis

10.1 Goals

Botulinum toxin can be used as a treatment for strabismus to improve eye alignment and promote binocularity.

10.2 Advantages

- Less invasive procedure which preserves the extraocular muscles for later surgery if needed and for patients at risk of developing anterior segment ischemia.
- Shorter procedure time, and as with incisional strabismus surgery, botulinum toxin injection in children requires general anesthesia but of significantly shorter duration.[1]
- The weakened muscle is not disinserted, reducing the risk of anterior segment ischemia.
- Can be used as a surgical treatment option for strabismus that is significantly variable or difficult to measure, with the understanding that incisional strabismus surgery may eventually be needed. The strabismus can thus be surgically managed earlier without the need for consistent measurements, as opposed to repeating the preoperative measurements multiple times and delaying surgery. Simultaneously, the potential for fusion can be assessed postoperatively.
- For some patients, the need for incisional surgery may be eliminated if strabismus does not recur.
- Lower risk of serious complications and possibly a lower risk of long-term overcorrections.[2]

10.3 Expectations

In the early postoperative period after botulinum toxin injection, overcorrection of the deviation and ptosis often occur,[2] which should be discussed in detail with the patient's family preoperatively, so that the family may anticipate these findings and be less alarmed if they occur. The ptosis can be expected to resolve as the strabismus improves.

10.4 Key Principles

- The mechanism of action of the toxin is at the neuromuscular junction where it blocks release of acetylcholine presynaptically. Paralysis of the muscle begins within 2 to 4 days and lasts for 8 to 12 weeks.
- While the effect of the toxin at the neuromuscular junction is transient, the injected muscle and its antagonist appear to undergo remodeling. Weakening of the injected muscle allows mild contracture of the antagonist muscle and, in turn, lengthening of the injected muscle, which persist even after the toxin is no longer in effect.
- In addition, taking advantage of the central drive for fusion, treatment with botulinum toxin to improve the eye alignment during the period of visual development in early childhood may promote the likelihood of a stable, long-term outcome.
- The use of botulinum toxin is more dependent on the potential for fusion than incisional strabismus surgery to improve and stabilize the eye alignment.
- The greater the volume of toxin that is injected, the higher the risk of adverse effects, specifically ptosis and spreading to other extraocular muscles, although they are transient. Larger volumes injected directly into the muscle may also result in more discomfort for patients.

10.5 Indications

Botulinum toxin has been used as a treatment for strabismus since the 1970s[3] and was approved by the Food and Drug Administration (FDA) in 1989 for the treatment of strabismus.[4] Botulinum toxin injection has been primarily reported as a treatment for various types of esotropia:

- Moderate-angle esotropia of 20 to 35 prism diopters (PD) with potential for fusion, including infantile esotropia,[5] acute comitant esotropia,[1] and cyclic esotropia.[6]
- Augmentation of medial rectus recessions in large angle esotropia greater than 50 to 60 PD

for which recessions greater than 6.0 to 6.5 mm of the medial rectus muscles may increase the risk of overcorrection in the future.

- In an acute abducens nerve palsy, weakening of the antagonist medial rectus muscle to reduce contracture of the medial rectus and to aid in the treatment of amblyopia in children while monitoring for recovery of the abducens nerve.[4]
- Weakening of the ipsilateral medial rectus muscle during a transposition procedure for an abducens nerve palsy or esotropic Duane syndrome to preserve the medial rectus muscle and decrease the risk of anterior segment ischemia.[7]

Other reported types of strabismus and scenarios in which botulinum toxin injection may be beneficial include:

- Residual strabismus or overcorrections, especially if intermittent, after prior surgery.[8]
- Partially accommodative esotropia[9] and esotropia in patients with cerebral palsy.[10]
- Patients with variable measurements or who are difficult to measure reliably may also be considered as candidates for treatment with botulinum toxin injection.

10.6 Contraindications

- Botulinum toxin injection is less effective as a sole treatment in patients with large deviations greater than 40 PD and chronic paralytic strabismus.
- Also appears to be less effective for exodeviations.[5]
- Known poor potential for fusion may preclude a satisfactory response to botulinum toxin treatment for strabismus.

10.7 Preoperative Preparation

A complete sensorimotor examination is performed as described in Chapter 1.7 Preoperative Preparation. Currently, there are no standardized guidelines for determining the number of units to inject based on the angle of the deviation or the type of strabismus. The author uses the following general guidelines using onabotulinum toxin A:

- For each muscle, 5 units for 25 to 30 PD and 7.5 units for 35 to 40 PD.
- Smaller doses of 2.5 units and up to 10 units may be used for smaller and larger deviations respectively.

- For augmenting a medial rectus recession for patients with large angle esotropia (≥60 PD), 5 units are injected into each medial rectus muscle.
- For a complete abducens nerve palsy, 5 to 7.5 units may be injected into the ipsilateral medial rectus muscle. For a partial abducens nerve palsy, 2.5 to 3 units may be injected.

10.8 Operative Technique

Using anatomic landmarks with familiarity of the path of the extraocular muscles posteriorly from their insertions, botulinum toxin injections can be administered without electromyographic (EMG) assistance, as general anesthetic agents suppress EMG activity and render it unreliable.

1. Reconstitute a vial of onabotulinum toxin A with 0.9% sterile sodium chloride saline and gently mix. See Tips and Pearls for the volume of saline to use.
2. Draw the volume with the predetermined number of units to be injected into a 1 mL TB syringe with an 18-gauge needle. Draw a small additional volume of approximately 0.75 mL into the TB syringe, so that the needle for injection can be primed.
3. Place a 1.5 inch 27-gauge needle onto the TB syringe and prime the needle, then recheck the volume in the syringe. If more than one muscle is to be injected, separate TB syringes with 1.5 inch 27-gauge needles can be prepared for each muscle prior to starting the procedure.
4. The patient is supine under general anesthesia. Phenylephrine 2.5% is instilled for vasoconstriction of the conjunctival vessels to decrease the risk of subconjunctival hemorrhage and to better visualize the anterior ciliary vessels on the muscle to be injected.
5. An eyelid speculum is placed and one drop of proparacaine, followed by one drop of 5% betadine, may be instilled.
6. For injection of a medial rectus muscle, the eye is abducted with toothed forceps. A second pair of forceps may be used to grasp the muscle through the conjunctiva to confirm the site of injection.
7. With the bevel of the needle facing down toward the muscle, pierce the conjunctiva just temporal to the plica semilunaris (▸ Fig. 10.1). The hand that is holding the needle is supported on the patient's face.

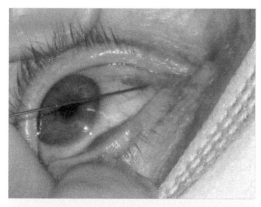

Fig. 10.1 With the bevel of the needle facing down toward the muscle, pierce the conjunctiva just temporal to the plica semilunaris, directing the needle so that it follows the approximate path of the medial rectus muscle.

8. The needle is advanced approximately 2 cm, following the direction of the medial rectus muscle slightly posteriorly until the tip of the needle just reaches the medial orbital wall, and is then pulled back slightly.
9. With the needle in stable position, the entire prepared volume of botulinum toxin in the TB syringe is injected into the muscle.
10. The head of the bed is then elevated for 1 to 2 minutes to try to decrease the risk of the toxin migrating toward the orbicularis, thereby decreasing the risk of ptosis.[1]
11. If an additional muscle is to be injected, the head of the bed is flattened, and the steps are repeated.

10.9 Tips and Pearls

- Reconstituting the botulinum toxin to a higher concentration (units per mL) may decrease the risk of ptosis or inadvertently affecting other extraocular muscles. By using a higher concentration of toxin, less volume of fluid is injected, which may be less likely to spread beyond the injected muscle.[5] A 100-unit vial of onabotulinum toxin A can be reconstituted with 1 mL of 0.9% sterile sodium chloride saline, for a concentration of 5 units per 0.05 mL. If 10 units are to be injected, the vial can be reconstituted with 0.5 mL for a concentration of 10 units per 0.05 mL.
- Onabotulinum toxin A is typically used for the treatment of strabismus. Other formulations of

botulinum toxin are available but notably do not have 1-to-1 equivalent therapeutic effects.[5]

10.10 What to Avoid

- Corneal irritation or abrasion.
- Subconjunctival hemorrhage.
- Inadvertent injection or spread into an adjacent muscle.
- Injury to the globe.

10.11 Complications

- There may be a higher risk of strabismus recurrence and need for reoperations after treatment with botulinum toxin injection, although the evidence for this is not yet conclusive. Recurrences may be treated with repeat botulinum toxin injections or with incisional strabismus surgery.[8,11]
- Ptosis and overcorrection are likely to occur in the early postoperative period, which is discussed in detail preoperatively.
- Perforation of the globe due to the proximity of the needle to the eye is also a potential but unlikely complication.

10.12 Postoperative Care

In most cases, postoperative medication is not needed, given the mild trauma to tissue that occurs with the injection. An antibiotic–steroid combination eyedrop may be used for 1 week following botulinum toxin injection if preferred.

References

[1] Wan MJ, Mantagos IS, Shah AS, Kazlas M, Hunter DG. Comparison of botulinum toxin with surgery for the treatment of acute-onset comitant esotropia in children. Am J Ophthalmol. 2017; 176:33–39

[2] Mahan M, Engel JM. The resurgence of botulinum toxin injection for strabismus in children. Curr Opin Ophthalmol. 2017; 28(5):460–464

[3] Scott AB. Botulinum toxin injection into extraocular muscles as an alternative to strabismus surgery. Ophthalmology. 1980; 87(10):1044–1049

[4] Escuder AG, Hunter DG. The role of botulinum toxin in the treatment of strabismus. Semin Ophthalmol. 2019; 34(4): 198–204

[5] de Alba Campomanes AG, Binenbaum G, Campomanes Eguiarte G. Comparison of botulinum toxin with surgery as primary treatment for infantile esotropia. J AAPOS. 2010; 14 (2):111–116

[6] Akyuz Unsal AI, Özkan SB, Ziylan S. Role of botulinum toxin type A in cyclic esotropia: a long-term follow-up. J Pediatr Ophthalmol Strabismus. 2019; 56(6):360–364

[7] Rosenbaum AL, Kushner BJ, Kirschen D. Vertical rectus muscle transposition and botulinum toxin (Oculinum) to medial rectus for abducens palsy. Arch Ophthalmol. 1989; 107(6):820–823

[8] Couser NL, Lambert SR. Botulinum toxin a treatment of consecutive esotropia in children. Strabismus. 2012; 20(4): 158–161

[9] Flores-Reyes EM, Castillo-López MG, Toledo-Silva R, Vargas-Ortega J, Murillo-Correa CE, Aguilar-Ruiz A. Botulinum toxin type A as treatment of partially accommodative esotropia. Arch Soc Esp Oftalmol. 2016; 91(3):120–124

[10] Petrushkin H, Oyewole K, Jain S. Botulinum toxin for the treatment of early-onset esotropia in children with cerebral palsy. J Pediatr Ophthalmol Strabismus. 2012; 49(2):125

[11] Leffler CT, Vaziri K, Schwartz SG, et al. Rates of reoperation and abnormal binocularity following strabismus surgery in children. Am J Ophthalmol. 2016; 162:159–166.e9

Section II

Orbital Procedures

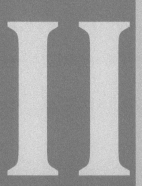

11 Nasolacrimal Duct Probing, Intubation, and Balloon Dilation

Catherine S. Choi and Maanasa Indaram

Summary
The vast majority of congenital nasolacrimal duct obstruction (NLDO) cases resolve by 1 year of age without intervention. For those with persistent NLDO, probing of the nasolacrimal system may be performed. This chapter discusses the relevant anatomy of the lacrimal drainage system and naso-lacrimal duct procedures to treat congenital NLDO, which generally have a high success rate.

NLDO manifests as tearing starting in early infancy with matting and crusting of the eyelashes, mucopurulent discharge, and recurrent episodes of conjunctivitis, eyelid edema and irritation. Most commonly, a membrane overlying the valve of Hasner at the junction of the distal nasolacrimal duct and the inferior meatus persists. Rarely, the puncta may be hypoplastic or even absent. Bony obstruction within the nasal cavity and lacrimal stones can also impede the flow of tears through the nasolacrimal duct. Some infants may develop a dacryocystocele which can become inflamed and infected (dacryocystitis), causing distention and presenting as an erythematous nodule inferior to the medial canthus.

Keywords: congenital nasolacrimal duct obstruction, dacryocystocele, nasolacrimal probing and irrigation, nasolacrimal intubation, balloon dacryoplasty

11.1 Goals

- Achieve normal flow of tears through the nasolacrimal system and alleviate obstructions in the nasolacrimal duct causing persistent tearing.
- Prevent dacryocystitis or recurrent conjunctivitis secondary to nasolacrimal duct obstruction (NLDO).
- Drain dacryocystoceles in neonates and young infants.
- Nasolacrimal duct intubation and balloon dacryoplasty are used to treat recurrent or persistent obstruction of the nasolacrimal duct.

11.2 Advantages

- Resolve symptomatic tearing which can cause local irritation and inflammation.

- Decrease the risk of dacryocystitis in neonates and young infants which can lead to sepsis in neonates due to an immature immune system.[5] In addition, bilateral dacryocystoceles may cause respiratory distress in neonates, requiring urgent surgical management.
- Nasolacrimal duct intubation and balloon dacryoplasty are advantageous procedures in children for whom treatment with probing alone has failed, in older children, and in children with Down syndrome or craniofacial anomalies.[2]

11.3 Expectations

- Congenital nasolacrimal duct obstruction (NLDO) occurs in approximately 5% of normal newborns.[3,5]
- Ninety percent of congenital NLDO cases resolve spontaneously within the first year of life.[1] The patient's family may attempt massage of the nasolacrimal duct to encourage resolution of persistent symptoms before considering surgical intervention. Proper nasolacrimal duct massage technique should be demonstrated to the family, including the appropriate amount of pressure to be used.
- Probing alone is successful in 75 to 90% of patients 6 to 36 months old.[5,6] The success rate of probing likely declines after 36 months, and intubation may be considered as the primary procedure.
- Dacryocystoceles may require nasal endoscopy in coordination with otorhinolaryngology to marsupialize the cyst.[7]
- If a stent is placed, complete resolution following stent removal occurs in approximately 90% of patients less than 4 years of age.[8] Persistent epiphora may occur while the stent is in place postoperatively.
- Nasolacrimal duct intubation and balloon dacryoplasty have similar success rates.[9]
- Mild to moderate epistaxis may occur immediately following the procedure due to intranasal manipulation.
- Long-term relief from tearing and irritation is expected, but sometimes it takes up to 2 weeks after surgery to achieve symptom resolution.

11.4 Key Principles

Understanding of lacrimal drainage system anatomy and use of the proper instruments improve the likelihood of uncomplicated and successful treatment in the majority of uncomplicated cases.

11.4.1 Anatomy

Tear drainage begins at the puncta (▶ Fig. 11.1). The upper and lower eyelids each contain a punctum medially which is 5 mm from the canthal angle superiorly and 6 mm from the canthal angle inferiorly.[10] Each punctum drains into a canaliculus which travels vertically for 2 mm, then horizontally for 8 mm. The superior and inferior canaliculi fuse to create a common canaliculus in 90% of patients. The canalicular structure empties into the lacrimal sac, which is 1.2 to 1.5 cm in length in the lacrimal sac fossa. The valve of Rosenmüller is a fold of tissue that serves as a one-way valve, helping to prevent tear reflux from the lacrimal sac into the canaliculus. The lacrimal sac then transitions into the nasolacrimal duct, which travels approximately 1.2 cm through the lacrimal canal and empties into the nasal cavity via the inferior meatus. The valve of Hasner is located just at the opening to the inferior meatus, helping to prevent reflux, and is a common site of obstruction in congenital NLDO.

11.5 Indications

- Persistent and symptomatic tearing from NLDO, especially beyond 1 year of age or if causing recurrent infections.
- Nonresolving or recurrent dacryocystocele with or without dacryocystitis or causing respiratory distress.
- Nasolacrimal duct probing with intubation or balloon dacryoplasty is considered in the following[2,5,11]:
  - Failed response to probing alone.
  - Children older than 3 to 4 years of age, as probing alone has a success rate of only 56%.[1,8]
  - Patients with suspected atypical anatomy, such as patients with Down syndrome or craniofacial anomalies, due to a higher risk of failure with probing and irrigation alone.[11]
  - If severe stenosis is encountered at the time of probing.

11.6 Contraindications

- Infants and children with acute dacryocystitis are treated with antibiotics for at least 48 hours prior to surgical management.
- Epiphora not caused by NLDO; for example, ocular surface disease, eyelid anomalies, and glaucoma.

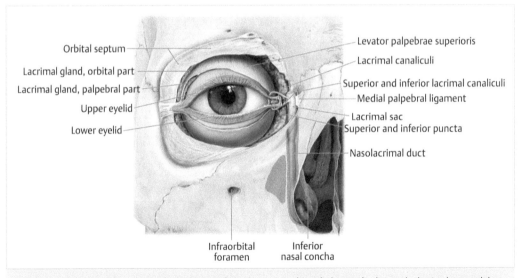

Fig. 11.1 The anatomy of nasolacrimal tear drainage from the puncta, through the canaliculi, into the lacrimal sac, and down through the nasolacrimal duct, emptying into the inferior meatus. (Reproduced with permission from Schünke M, Schulte E, Schumacher U. Thieme Atlas of Anatomy: Head, Neck and Neuroanatomy, 2nd edition. Stuttgart: Thieme; 2016.)

- Agenesis of the puncta, canaliculi, or proximal lacrimal drainage system requires an alternative approach such as eyelid cut-down and/or conjunctivodacryocystorhinostomy and should be referred to an oculoplastic surgeon.
- Bony distal obstruction of the nasolacrimal duct may require dacryocystorhinostomy or endonasal surgery.
- Nasolacrimal fistula to the external skin, which requires complete excision of the fistula.

11.7 Preoperative Preparation

- A complete eye exam should be performed to rule out other causes of epiphora.
- Evaluate the periorbital region and eyelids for any lesions or abnormalities of the puncta. The tear lake is also inspected, and a dye disappearance test can be helpful to confirm the diagnosis of NLDO.
- The surgeon should discuss the expectations following surgery, including persistent epiphora in the early postoperative period or while a stent is in place. The risk of failure with the possible need for further surgery is also discussed.
- Discuss management of the airway with the anesthesia team, as nasal irrigation and bleeding can cause laryngospasm or other airway obstruction. Although nasolacrimal probing and irrigation is typically brief and can be performed with mask sedation or a laryngeal mask airway, endotracheal intubation better secures the airway, especially for longer cases with stent placement or balloon dacryoplasty.
- Nasolacrimal duct procedures are classified as clean procedures and are not sterile. Gentle pressure may be applied over the nasolacrimal sac inferior to the medial canthus to express and remove purulent material through the puncta before starting the procedure. The surgical field is then prepped with gauze and cotton-tip applicators soaked in 5% betadine to clean the eyelids and eyelashes, and sterile towels can be placed around the surgical field.

11.8 Operative Technique

11.8.1 Nasolacrimal Duct Probing with or without Irrigation

1. Both the upper and lower puncta are examined. Occasionally, a membrane may be visualized over either or both puncta, which can be gently opened using a punctal dilator before proceeding with the remainder of the procedure.
2. Probing through the upper punctum may result in less trauma to the proximal canalicular system with lower risk of false passage creation.[12] However, if the patient's anatomy precludes easy passage of the nasolacrimal probe through the upper canalicular system, the lower punctum and canalicular system are probed for the procedure.
3. The upper eyelid is gently everted to visualize the upper punctum. The smallest available punctal dilator is inserted into the punctum, perpendicular to the eyelid margin to dilate the punctum (▶ Fig. 11.2). Lateral traction is placed on the eyelid, and the dilator is redirected and advanced medially while rotating it along its long axis to dilate the proximal canalicular system. When performing this procedure for congenital dacryocystoceles, dilation of the canaliculus can help

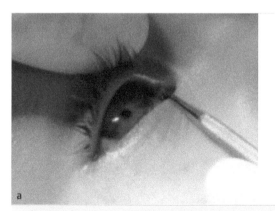
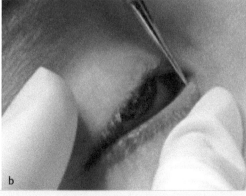

Fig. 11.2 A punctal dilator is used to dilate the **(a)** upper and **(b)** lower puncta.

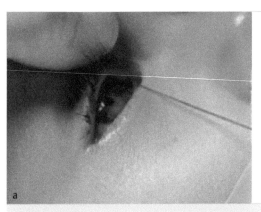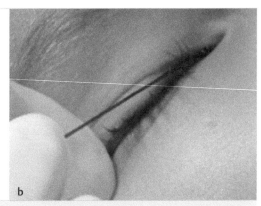

Fig. 11.3 A #00 Bowman probe is inserted into the upper punctum **(a)** perpendicular to the eyelid margin and **(b)** then redirected nasally and advanced into the lacrimal sac to a firm, bony stop.

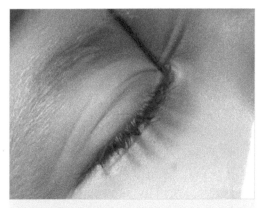

Fig. 11.4 Once the Bowman probe reaches a bony stop, the lateral tension on the eyelid is released, and the probe is redirected inferiorly, posteriorly, and slightly laterally into the nasolacrimal duct.

decompress the dacryocystocele, making the remainder of the procedure easier to perform.[12]

4. The punctal dilator is removed, and a #000 or #00 Bowman probe is inserted into the upper punctum perpendicular to the eyelid margin for 1 to 2 mm (► Fig. 11.3a), then directed nasally into the upper canaliculus and then the lacrimal sac while simultaneously placing lateral traction on the eyelid to straighten the canaliculus. The probe should slide easily through the proximal canalicular system and then reach a firm, bony stop with no soft tissue palpable to decrease the risk of creating a false passage (► Fig. 11.3b). Note that a smaller Bowman probe (#000) may be needed for probing of congenital dacryocystoceles, although Bowman probes smaller than #00 may increase the risk of false passage creation.

5. Once the Bowman probe is confirmed to be abutting bone, it is rotated sharply 90 degrees and then advanced inferiorly, posteriorly, and slightly laterally through the lacrimal sac and nasolacrimal duct into the nasal cavity (► Fig. 11.4). The tension on the eyelid is also released to prevent tearing of the punctum as the Bowman probe is advanced. In some cases, a popping sensation can be felt as the probe passes through the membrane at the valve of Hasner. In other cases, significant stenosis of the bony portion of the nasolacrimal duct may require additional gentle pressure to allow passage of the probe. Once the Bowman probe has been advanced, a second Bowman probe of any size can be held externally over the nose and lined up with the Bowman probe in the nasolacrimal system to gauge the position of the distal end of the probe in the nasal cavity. If probing for a congenital dacryocystocele in the office without sedation, elevate the infant's head once the popping sensation is felt to allow the infant to swallow the fluid that was filling the cyst without aspirating.[12]

6. Larger diameter Bowman probes, up to #0 or #1, can be used to probe the lacrimal drainage system in a similar manner.

7. A large #7 or #8 Bowman probe can then be used to verify the presence of the smaller Bowman probe in the ipsilateral nasal cavity by sliding the larger probe under the inferior turbinate and feeling for metal-on-metal contact, as well as observing movement of the smaller Bowman probe when it is in contact with the large probe (► Fig. 11.5). The Bowman probe can also be directly visualized in some

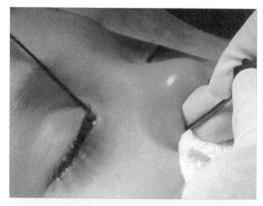

Fig. 11.5 Verification of the Bowman probe within the nasal cavity using a #7 or #8 Bowman probe by metal-on-metal contact.

cases by placing a nasal speculum in the nasal cavity or by nasal endoscopy if available.

8. The Bowman probe in the nasolacrimal system is then removed, and the above steps may be repeated for the lower punctum and canaliculus.

9. To verify patency of the nasolacrimal system following probing, fluorescein-stained saline can be irrigated through the upper punctum with a 23-gauge cannula attached to a 3 mL syringe. The cannula is advanced and the nasolacrimal system is irrigated. The opposite punctum may simultaneously be occluded with a punctal dilator or by manual pressure using a cotton-tip applicator to prevent reflux. The fluorescein-stained saline is recovered from the naris with an 8-French suction catheter.

11.8.2 Nasolacrimal Duct Probing with Intubation

There are several insertion systems and stents available for intubation of the nasolacrimal system. Monocanalicular or bicanalicular stents can be placed using Ritleng, Crawford, or Masterka systems as per the surgeon's preference and surgical center availability.[2,12,13,14] The authors' preference is to use the Ritleng system to insert a monocanalicular stent due to ease of placement and removal without the need for securing a knot in the nose as required for bicanalicular stents. The Ritleng system for intubation is comprised of a hollow probe with a groove and a monocanalicular or bicanalicular silicone stent with an attached polypropylene suture, which is thicker at its end than where it is bonded to the stent:

1. After induction of anesthesia, small pledgets soaked with oxymetazoline hydrochloride 0.05% may be placed into the ipsilateral naris with bayonet forceps for vasoconstriction of the nasal mucosa to reduce intra- and postoperative bleeding.

2. Steps 1 to 8 of Chapter 11.8.1 Nasolacrimal Duct Probing with or without Irrigation are then performed. The pledgets can be removed before any probes are introduced.

3. The Ritleng probe with or without the stylet in place is passed into the nasolacrimal system through the punctum in a similar manner as a Bowman probe. It is essential to confirm the location of the Ritleng probe in the nose with *metal-to-metal* contact before proceeding with the procedure to ensure that the stent will be recovered in the naris. The stylet is then removed.

4. A monocanalicular or bicanalicular stent with attached suture is inserted into the hollow Ritleng probe, which is rotated for the groove to be facing anteriorly. The suture is carefully advanced through the probe with nontoothed forceps, a few millimeters at a time, to prevent inadvertent kinking of the suture as it is passed, which would make its retrieval through the nose more difficult.

5. As the suture is advanced into the nose, it usually exits the naris on its own but may remain coiled in the nose, in which case a Ritleng hook can be inserted to retrieve the suture from under the inferior turbinate. Once the suture is out of the naris, the Ritleng probe is removed, keeping the stent in place:

   a) If a monocanalicular stent is used, the suture is gently pulled through the nose, allowing the stent to pass through the nasolacrimal system, until the proximal end of the stent, which has a collarette, is securely seated over the punctum. The authors recommend inserting the stent through the upper punctum, which renders the stent more difficult to remove prematurely by the patient. The distal end of the stent is gently tugged from the naris and held taut. It is then trimmed just inside the naris to ensure that it will not be felt by the patient and potentially pulled, but also so that it does not retract into the nasolacrimal duct and no longer bridges the valve of Hasner (▶ Fig. 11.6).

   b) If a bicanalicular stent is used, steps 3 to 5 are performed with the Ritleng probe through both the upper and lower puncta. The suture

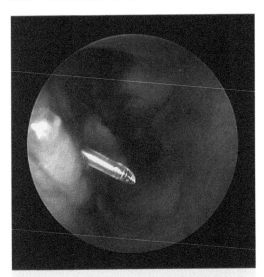

Fig. 11.6 Trimmed silicone stent under the inferior turbinate on nasal endoscopy. (Reproduced with permission from Freitag S, Lefebvre D, Lee N, et al, eds. Ophthalmic Plastic Surgery: Tricks of the Trade, 1st edition. Stuttgart: Thieme; 2019.)

ends are then trimmed from the stent. Both ends of the stent are gently tugged from the naris and tied with a 1–1 throw square knot over a needle holder, ensuring that there is appropriate tension to avoid early extrusion of the stent but without excessive traction on the proximal canalicular system.[12] The knot should be small so that it can be safely pulled through the nasolacrimal system during removal. The ends of the silicone stent are then trimmed just inside the naris. The knot should retract into the nose so that the distal end is not felt by the patient and potentially pulled, but the stent should bridge the valve of Hasner.

6. Stents are recommended to be kept in place for 3 to 4 months to decrease the risk of recurrence.[12,15] Stent removal occurs in the office setting with the help of a family member and without sedation in the majority of cases. A topical anesthetic is instilled.
   a) Monocanalicular stents can be removed by using nontoothed forceps to grasp the collarette of the stent at the punctum and then pull it out completely.
   b) Bicanalicular stents are removed by pulling the loop of the stent between the upper and lower puncta with nontoothed forceps and cutting the loop. Using the forceps, the stent is removed through either punctum, as long as a

small square knot was tied. If there is resistance as the stent is being removed, direct visualization such as with nasal endoscopy may be needed to remove the stent through the nose. If the patient requires sedation for removal, and the stent is not easily removed through the punctum or by direct visualization of the nasal cavity, an alternative method is to use a very thin Bowman probe which is inserted into the cut end of the loop at the upper punctum, passed through the nasolacrimal system, and then accessed in the nasal cavity with the stent which can then be removed.[16]

11.8.3 Nasolacrimal Duct Probing with Balloon Dilation

1. Steps 1 to 8 of *Nasolacrimal Duct Probing without Irrigation* are first performed. Intravenous dexamethasone may be given intraoperatively.
2. The inflation protocol, as specified by the manufacturer in the labeling of the selected product, is then followed as described below.
3. A semiflexible wire catheter with an inflatable balloon at the tip is lubricated, and the inflation apparatus, which has a manometer and locking mechanism, is primed with balanced salt solution.
4. The catheter is introduced into the upper canalicular system and advanced into the nasal cavity in a similar manner as a Bowman probe. The distal position of the catheter can be confirmed by direct visualization or by carefully grasping the catheter with nontoothed forceps in the nose and gently moving it side to side.
5. The inflation apparatus is then attached to the catheter. With the 15-mm marking on the catheter at the punctum, which positions the balloon at the level of the valve of Hasner, the balloon is inflated until the manometer reaches 8 atmospheres of pressure, which is maintained for 90 seconds (▶ Fig. 11.7). The inflated balloon should securely remain in position with gentle tugging on the tube. Easy slippage or inability to maintain 8 atmospheres of pressure may indicate balloon leakage, and the catheter should be replaced. After 90 seconds, the balloon is deflated and then inflated again to 8 atmospheres for 60 more seconds, then deflated again.[17]
6. The catheter is withdrawn 5 mm to the 10-mm marking, which positions the balloon at the level of the nasolacrimal duct. Again, the balloon is inflated until the manometer reaches

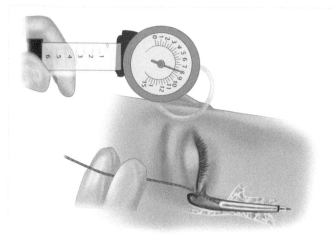

Fig. 11.7 The balloon is positioned at the level of the valve of Hasner and inflated until the manometer reaches 8 atmospheres of pressure.

8 atmospheres of pressure, which is maintained for 90 seconds. After 90 seconds, the balloon is deflated and then inflated again to 8 atmospheres for 60 more seconds, then completely deflated.

7. The deflated catheter is then carefully removed while rotating the catheter as it is withdrawn to minimize trauma to the surrounding tissues.

8. Fluorescein-stained saline can then be irrigated through the upper or lower punctum with a 23-gauge cannula attached to a 3-mL syringe. The cannula is advanced and the nasolacrimal system is irrigated. The opposite punctum may simultaneously be occluded with a punctal dilator to avoid reflux. The fluorescein-stained saline is then recovered from the nose with an 8-French suction catheter.

11.9 Tips and Pearls

- Recall that the vertical portion of the canaliculus is only 1 to 2 mm in length during insertion of the punctal dilator and Bowman probes.
- Ophthalmic ointment may be used for lubrication on the Bowman probes prior to insertion.
- During insertion of the punctal dilator and Bowman probes, lateral traction applied to the eyelid to straighten the canaliculus allows for smoother passage of the instrument and decreases the risk of injury to the canaliculus or false passage creation. It is also helpful to angle the probe toward the medial canthus: slightly inferiorly when passing through the upper punctum and slightly superiorly when passing through the lower punctum. If there is any soft tissue restriction,

the probe should not be forced past the area of restriction and should instead be retracted and repositioned.

- Palpation of a definite bony stop with the Bowman probe is a key step to avoid creation of a false passage. Then, as the probe is rotated, care should be taken to avoid inadvertently shifting the Bowman probe out of the nasolacrimal system by holding the opposite end of the probe against the brow. Once the probe is rotated inferiorly, it should glide along the nasolacrimal duct.
- The Bowman probe should not be advanced too far into the nasal cavity so that it becomes embedded in the floor of the nose or even penetrates the palate.
- To achieve metal-to-metal contact, insert the larger probe by entering along the nasal floor to slide under the inferior turbinate, and then sliding it laterally to meet the smaller probe in the nose.
- When performing metal-to-metal contact, if it is felt that the space under the inferior turbinate is tight, inferior turbinate infracture toward the nasal septum can be performed. A Freer elevator is positioned by sliding it along the lateral nasal wall. Once it is under the inferior turbinate, it is pushed medially with steady pressure on the inferior turbinate to displace it medially. A small "crack" or release should be felt.
- Probing a dacryocystocele in a neonate may be performed without anesthesia by swaddling the infant and using a pacifier with sugar water for comfort. This may be preferred by some families due to concerns about risks of anesthesia during infancy. Dilation of the canaliculus alone may partially decompress the dacryocystocele, and

then a small Bowman probe (#000) is used with gentle pressure to guide the probe along the nasolacrimal system. Because recurrence of dacryocystoceles that appear to self-resolve with massage or after probing alone is not uncommon, the family may be given the option for the patient to undergo probing under anesthesia with nasal endoscopy and marsupialization of the cyst, in coordination with otorhinolaryngology.

- If probing does not resolve the NLDO, it may be beneficial to coordinate a secondary procedure with otorhinolaryngology for concurrent nasal endoscopy.

11.9.1 Nasolacrimal Duct Probing with Intubation

- If the Ritleng hook is needed to retrieve the stent from the naris, the hook is inserted flat with its open end facing the nasal septum. When metal-to-metal contact with the Ritleng probe is achieved, the hook is rotated 180 degrees to capture the suture.
- The monocanalicular stent is available in two collarette sizes: 3 and 4 mm. The smaller size can be used for infants and young children.
- If placing a monocanalicular stent, avoid overdilating the punctum, so that the punctal anchor on the collarette will fit snugly in the punctum.
- When placing a monocanalicular stent, ensure that the collarette lies completely flat over the punctum so that the patient does not feel the stent, which may result in the patient pulling or rubbing the stent out of position. A punctal dilator can be used to push the center of the collarette into the punctum to secure its position.
- After placing and tying a bicanalicular stent with a small 1–1 throw square knot, the knot can be sutured to the mucosa of the lateral nasal wall with 4–0 chromic gut suture on a small half-circle needle to decrease the risk of early extrusion.

11.9.2 Nasolacrimal Duct Probing with Balloon Dilation

- For balloon dilation, the 3-mm lacrimal catheter is typically used for patients older than 2 years of age, while the smaller 2-mm catheter is used for younger patients.

11.10 What to Avoid

- Creation of a false passage can result in an unsuccessful procedure and development of scarring that can complicate future surgeries if tearing persists.
  - Avoid passing the Bowman probe with excessive force through the nasolacrimal system. Attempting to push the probe through soft tissue resistance increases the risk of false passage creation proximally.
  - Rotating the Bowman probe before a definite bony stop increases the risk of false passage creation distally.
- Avoid excessive manipulation within the nasal cavity which can result in significant bleeding, making the procedure more challenging and possibly affecting the airway, if mask anesthesia or a laryngeal mask airway is used.

11.10.1 Nasolacrimal Duct Probing with Intubation

- Avoid passing the Ritleng hook into the nose multiple times when retrieving the suture from the nose.
- If the position of the Ritleng probe was not confirmed with metal-to-metal contact before the stent was passed into the probe, it is possible that the nasolacrimal system was not yet patent or a false passage was created, especially if the stent cannot be retrieved in the nasal cavity. Otorhinolaryngology may be consulted to recover the stent by direct visualization with nasal endoscopy and possible mucosal cutdown if needed.

11.10.2 Nasolacrimal Duct Probing with Balloon Dilation

- Avoid damage to the canaliculus by ensuring that the balloon is not inadvertently pulled into the canaliculus and inflated.

11.11 Complications

- The primary risk of procedures for congenital NLDO is failure to respond or recurrence, in which case additional surgery can be offered. In rare cases, evaluation for dacryocystorhinostomy may be needed.
- Creation of a false passage, possibly with scar formation.

- Dacryocystitis or periorbital cellulitis requiring treatment with topical and systemic antibiotics.
- Mild-moderate epistaxis can be expected from the intranasal manipulation and can usually be addressed with gentle pressure and the use of intranasal vasoconstrictors. If the bleeding is severe, otorhinolaryngology is consulted for possible cauterization.
- Complications of monocanalicular stent placement include granuloma formation, corneal or conjunctival abrasions, intracanalicular migration of the stent, and early extrusion and loss of the stent.[16]
- Placement of a bicanalicular stent risks damaging or cheesewiring through the puncta, possibly due to a stent that is too tight or, in some cases, due to rapid growth of the child. Lateral extrusion of the loop at the puncta can also occur, causing anxiety for the family and usually resulting in early removal of the stent.
- Extrusion and removal of the stent before 3 to 4 months may result in procedure failure and recurrence of NLDO.
- With balloon dacryoplasty, the lack of an implanted stent theoretically decreases the risk of complications.[9]

11.12 Postoperative Care

- An antibiotic-corticosteroid combination eye drop or ointment is used for 1 week.
- The patient's family should be aware that mild epistaxis and blood-tinged tears may be present in the first 24 hours after the procedure. In addition, resolution of NLDO is typically not immediate. If a stent was inserted, symptoms may persist while the stent is in place.
- Patency of the nasolacrimal system may be confirmed postoperatively by repeating the dye disappearance test in the office.

References

[1] Wong RK, VanderVeen DK. Presentation and management of congenital dacryocystocele. Pediatrics. 2008; 122(5): e1108–e1112

[2] Napier ML, Armstrong DJ, McLoone SF, McLoone EM. Congenital nasolacrimal duct obstruction: comparison of two different treatment algorithms. J Pediatr Ophthalmol Strabismus. 2016; 53(5):285–291

[3] Petersen RA, Robb RM. The natural course of congenital obstruction of the nasolacrimal duct. J Pediatr Ophthalmol Strabismus. 1978; 15(4):246–250

[4] Frick KD, Hariharan L, Repka MX, Chandler D, Melia BM, Beck RW, Pediatric Eye Disease Investigator Group (PEDIG). Cost-effectiveness of 2 approaches to managing nasolacrimal duct obstruction in infants: the importance of the spontaneous resolution rate. Arch Ophthalmol. 2011; 129 (5):603–609

[5] Repka MX, Chandler DL, Beck RW, et al. Pediatric Eye Disease Investigator Group. Primary treatment of nasolacrimal duct obstruction with probing in children younger than 4 years. Ophthalmology. 2008; 115(3):577–584.e3

[6] Robb RM. Probing and irrigation for congenital nasolacrimal duct obstruction. Arch Ophthalmol. 1986; 104(3): 378–379

[7] Lueder GT. The association of neonatal dacryocystoceles and infantile dacryocystitis with nasolacrimal duct cysts (an American Ophthalmological Society thesis). Trans Am Ophthalmol Soc. 2012; 110:74–93

[8] Repka MX, Chandler DL, Holmes JM, et al. Pediatric Eye Disease Investigator Group. Balloon catheter dilation and nasolacrimal duct intubation for treatment of nasolacrimal duct obstruction after failed probing. Arch Ophthalmol. 2009; 127 (5):633–639

[9] Repka MX, Melia BM, Beck RW, et al. Pediatric Eye Disease Investigator Group. Primary treatment of nasolacrimal duct obstruction with nasolacrimal duct intubation in children younger than 4 years of age. J AAPOS. 2008; 12(5): 445–450

[10] Dutton JJ. Surgical anatomy of the lacrimal drainage system. In: Atlas of Oculoplastic and Orbital Surgery. 2nd ed. Philadelphia, PA: Wolters Kluwer; 2019:243–247

[11] Casady DR, Meyer DR, Simon JW, Stasior GO, Zobal-Ratner JL. Stepwise treatment paradigm for congenital nasolacrimal duct obstruction. Ophthal Plast Reconstr Surg. 2006; 22(4): 243–247

[12] Montagos I. Probing, irrigation, and intubation in congenital nasolacrimal duct obstruction. In: Freitag SK, Lee NG, Lefebvre DR, Yoon MK, eds. Ophthalmic Plastic Surgery: Tricks of the Trade. New York, NY: Thieme; 2020:160–164

[13] Khatib L, Nazemzadeh M, Revere K, Katowitz WR, Katowitz JA. Use of the Masterka for complex nasolacrimal duct obstruction in children. J AAPOS. 2017; 21(5):380–383

[14] Eustis HS, Nguyen AH. The treatment of congenital nasolacrimal duct obstruction in children: a retrospective review. J Pediatr Ophthalmol Strabismus. 2018; 55(1):65–67

[15] Dotan G, Nelson LB. Congenital nasolacrimal duct obstruction: common management policies among pediatric ophthalmologists. J Pediatr Ophthalmol Strabismus. 2015; 52(1): 14–19

[16] Katowitz WR, Nazemzadeh M, Katowitz JA. Initial management of pediatric lower system problems: probing and silicone stents and balloons. In: Katowitz JA, Katowitz WR, eds. Pediatric Oculoplastic Surgery. 2nd ed. Cham, Switzerland: Springer; New York, NY: Thieme; 2018:479–500

[17] Wladis EJ, Aakalu VK, Yen MT, Bilyk JR, Sobel RK, Mawn LA. Balloon dacryoplasty for congenital nasolacrimal duct obstruction: a report by the American Academy of Ophthalmology. Ophthalmology. 2018; 125:1654–1657

12 Dermoid Cyst Excision

Alison B. Callahan

Summary

Dermoid cysts are benign choristomas which are present at birth and continue to enlarge commensurate with a child's natural growth. This chapter will discuss excision of the more common superficial dermoid cyst.

Keywords: dermoid cyst, choristoma, dumbbell-type dermoid, orbital granulomatous inflammation

12.1 Goals

The goal of this procedure is to remove the lesion and to do so completely. To remove the lesion in its entirety, care is taken to keep the cyst wall intact throughout the procedure, with its contents contained within its capsule. Removal of the lesion completely avoids the possibility of further growth and future recurrences as well as postoperative orbital granulomatous inflammation (a sequela of ruptured contents described below).[1,2] Although removal of the lesion is the primary goal, a secondary goal of the procedure is to eliminate an often-noticeable deformity and to optimize and minimize the incision utilized for excision. Usually a segmental upper eyelid crease incision is utilized to access the lesion, although a sub-brow incision can also be used for much larger or more adherent lesions.

12.2 Advantages

Although dermoid cysts are benign lesions, the material contained within them can cause severe inflammation. This material is kept at bay by its natural encapsulation, but even mild trauma such as a bumped head or unintentional fall of a newly walking toddler can cause a rupture. As the content leaks or spills out into adjacent tissue, it can cause a significant granulomatous inflammation, often mimicking the appearance of periocular cellulitis. Additionally, uncontrolled rupture can disseminate contents subcutaneously, rendering future complete excision surgically challenging. To avoid the possibility of future inflammation and maximize the ease of complete excision, it is generally recommended to remove these choristomas at a relatively young age. Although there is no absolute age, standard of care is usually to remove them around the age of 1 year old—beyond the period of higher risk general anesthesia in infancy and before fully ambulatory and at greater risk of accidental trauma. By removing the lesion at a relatively young age, it also minimizes the size of the incision required for excision and eliminates future molding of surrounding tissues that can occur with untouched, chronic lesions.

12.3 Expectations

The expectation of dermoid excision is that the cyst is removed safely without complication or deformity.

12.4 Key Principles

Dermoid cysts are most frequently located in the superotemporal quadrant at the frontozygomatic suture line,[3] but can also occur at other suture lines including the superonasal frontoethmoidal suture line. Superficial dermoid cysts tend to present within the first year of life as a visible and/or palpable mass noted at the orbital rim.[1] Deep dermoid cysts grow innocuously within the orbit and consequently present later in life (teen or adult years) with manifestations such as proptosis or globe dystopia.[1] When approaching dermoid cyst excision, plan your approach and take it slowly. Utilize the most cosmetically favorable incision possible—often an upper eyelid crease incision. That being said, give yourself the access and exposure you need to successfully remove the lesion completely and do not compromise adequate exposure for a more cosmetically favorable incision. Without proper exposure, one risks intraoperative rupture which puts the patient at risk for recurrence and ongoing inflammation if not thoroughly debrided.

Use layer-by-layer dissection until the cyst is encountered and then dissect around the capsule with as much blunt dissection as possible and limited sharp dissection. Consider leaving a few fibers of tissue on the capsule to grasp for traction to avoid risking rupture by grasping the capsule itself. A cryotherapy probe can also be utilized and provides excellent traction without rupture when applied to the capsule.

Occasionally, the cystic cavity will extend through the lateral wall into the temporal fossa forming a "dumbbell"-shaped lesion. These lesions should be suspected preoperatively due to their immobility and confirmed with imaging. When excising this type of lesion, attempts should be made to eliminate components from the bony canal with a drill or bone curette and irrigation.

12.5 Indications

Presence of a slowly growing congenital lesion at the orbital rim, clinically and/or radiologically consistent with a dermoid cyst.

12.6 Contraindications

Patient families who do not desire surgical intervention for this benign lesion may decline excision. If surgery *is* planned, prior to embarking upon excision, one should have confidence in the presumed diagnosis. Lesions which are in any way atypical, including rapidly expanding lesions, lesions with a deeper discoloration or hue, or lesions in an atypical location, warrant imaging. Given that meningoencephaloceles also occur in the superonasal orbit, it is prudent to consider imaging for any medial dermoid. Immobile lesions suspicious for a dumbbell-type dermoid also warrant imaging.

It is preferable to remove an uninflamed lesion. Excising a recently ruptured dermoid often proves challenging for many reasons: the cyst wall or capsule is no longer a reliable surgical plane to follow, inflammation causes adherence of adjacent tissue as well as a significantly more vascular field with less visibility, and material has been cast into adjacent subcutaneous tissues. If a lesion has been recently ruptured or if there is active inflammation, one should defer excision until the area has quieted with time, often with a course of oral corticosteroids.

12.7 Preoperative Preparation

- Clinical evaluation of the lesion, including its size, location, mobility, and signs of active inflammation:
  - These factors inform timing of excision and planned surgical approach.
- Imaging, when clinically indicated:
  - Atypical lesions.
  - Medially located lesions.
  - Immobile lesions suspicious for dumbbell-type dermoid.
- Preoperative photography is recommended.
- The planned incision is marked with a marking pen (▶ Fig. 12.1) prior to infiltrating the tissue with approximately 1 mL of local anesthetic with epinephrine. The choice of anesthetic is per surgeon's preference; 1 to 2% lidocaine or 0.5% bupivacaine may be used with 1:200:000 epinephrine for vasoconstriction and hemostasis.

12.8 Operative Technique

1. The patient is prepped and draped in the usual sterile fashion for ophthalmic plastic surgery.
2. A #15 blade is used to make a skin incision along the previously made mark.
3. Hemostasis throughout the procedure is achieved with cautery.
4. The opposing skin-muscle edges are tented with toothed forceps, and the underlying orbicularis is incised with blunt Wescott scissors.
5. Layer-by-layer dissection posteriorly is conducted until the lesion is encountered (▶ Fig. 12.2).
6. With retraction of the skin incision, careful dissection utilizing blunt dissection whenever possible is carried out around the capsule.
7. Once the lesion is sufficiently liberated, it can usually be "rotated," "flipped," or "delivered" out of the incision and any remaining attachments dissected free (▶ Fig. 12.3).
8. The liberated lesion is sent for pathologic evaluation (▶ Fig. 12.4).

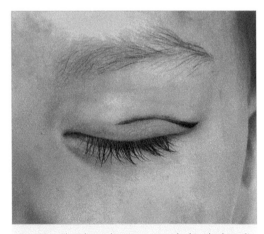

Fig. 12.1 The planned incision is marked in the lateral eyelid crease prior to infiltrating with lidocaine with epinephrine.

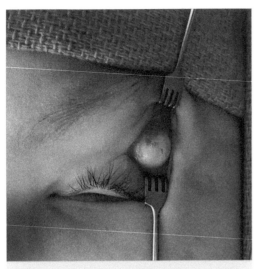

Fig. 12.2 The anterior surface of the dermoid cyst is visible following layer-by-layer dissection.

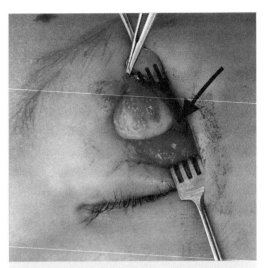

Fig. 12.3 After circumferential dissection, rotating the dermoid reveals residual posterior attachments (arrow). Note that a small amount of pericapsular tissue is left in place and grasped with forceps for traction without rupture.

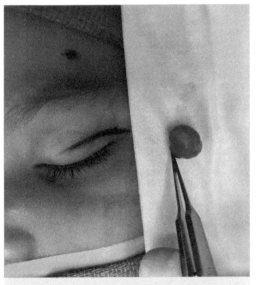

Fig. 12.4 The completely excised, unruptured dermoid cyst, which will be sent for pathologic evaluation.

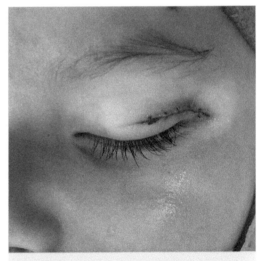

Fig. 12.5 The skin incision is closed with interrupted 6–0 plain gut suture. Note blanching of the skin at the surgical site from infiltration of epinephrine with the local anesthetic.

9. Hemostasis is confirmed prior to closing.
10. The skin edges are reapproximated and closed with interrupted absorbable suture such as 6–0 plain gut suture (▶ Fig. 12.5):

a) Deeply buried dermal sutures using 6–0 chromic gut suture may be needed for larger incisions in the brow.

12.9 Tips and Pearls

- Take your time.
- Counter-traction is key to reveal pericapsular attachments tethering the cyst:
  - Rotate the lesion to expose and tent various sides of the lesion for dissection.
- Choose your method of counter-traction wisely to avoid rupturing the lesion with forceps:
  - Leave a few fibers on the capsule to grasp and retract.
  - Consider utilizing a cryotherapy probe.
- If one area of pericapsular dissection is proving difficult, move to another; often, once one area is liberated, the lesion can be rotated or retracted in such a way to make the previously challenging area more accessible.
- For dumbbell-type dermoids, be prepared to evacuate the bony canal with a curette or drill.
- Although most lesions are well away from the frontal branch of the facial nerve (cranial nerve 7), be cognizant of the surgical site as it relates to the course of this nerve.
- Allow a recently ruptured dermoid to quiet down before excision.

12.10 What to Avoid

- Uncontrolled rupture.
- Incomplete removal.
- Facial nerve injury.

12.11 Complications

- Recurrence.
- Inflammation.
- Bleeding.
- Infection.
- Partial facial nerve palsy.

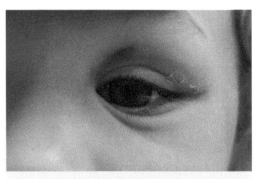

Fig. 12.6 Postoperatively, the wound is kept clean and dry, and ointment may be applied.

12.12 Postoperative Care

- Limit activity to the extent possible for approximately 1 week.
- Keep the wound clean and dry (▶ Fig. 12.6).
- Avoid submerging the head, e.g., swimming or bath tub, for 2 weeks.
- An ophthalmic antibiotic, corticosteroid, or nonmedicated ointment may be applied to the wound postoperatively.

References

[1] Katowitz WR, Fries PD, Kazim MK. Benign pediatric orbital tumors. In: Katowitz JA, Katowitz WR, eds. Pediatric Oculoplastic Surgery. 2nd ed. Cham, Switzerland: Springer; 2018:435–490

[2] White VA, Rootman JR. The pathologic basis of orbital disease. In: Rootman J, ed. Diseases of the Orbit: A Multidisciplinary Approach. 2nd ed. Philadelphia, PA: Lippincott Williams & Wilkins; 2003:121–167

[3] Dutton JJ, Sines DT, Elner VM. Orbital tumors. In: Black EH, Nesi FA, Gladstone G, Levine MR, Calvano CJ, eds. Smith and Nesi's Ophthalmic Plastic and Reconstructive Surgery. 3rd ed. New York: Springer; 2012:811–910

Section III

Anterior Segment Procedures

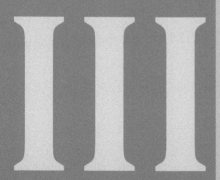

13 Pediatric Cataract Surgery

Sylvia H. Yoo

Summary

Infants and young children under 8 to 9 years of age who are born with or develop cataracts are at risk of developing deprivation amblyopia, which can result in severely decreased vision, depending on the size, location, and density of the lens opacity, age at onset, duration of visual deprivation, and whether the cataract is unilateral or bilateral. Timely intervention is crucial for the optimal treatment of infantile and juvenile cataracts. Cataract extraction is an early, critical step in the management of cataracts in the pediatric population, after which the treatment of amblyopia and monitoring for complications, including visual axis opacification and glaucoma, continue for years and are equally critical.

Keywords: infantile cataract, juvenile cataract, aspirationanterior vitrectomy, posterior capsulotomy, intraocular lens, aphakia, secondary intraocular lens, visual axis opacification

13.1 Goals

The goal of cataract surgery in infants and children is to clear the visual axis in an eye with visual deprivation causing amblyopia and then closely monitor and treat amblyopia and any complications that occur.

13.2 Advantages

Although nonsurgical treatments including pupillary dilation, correction of refractive error, and occlusion therapy may be used to treat small cataracts that appear "borderline" amblyogenic, cataract surgery is the sole treatment available to treat visual deprivation. Pupillary dilation with phenylephrine and tropicamide can be considered as a nonsurgical treatment option for small paracentral cataracts.[1] Cyclopentolate and atropine are avoided due the risk of anticholinergic side effects on the central nervous system in infants[2] and due to resulting cycloplegia. However, availability of phenylephrine and tropicamide eye drops on an outpatient basis is often limited, even when prescribed, and these drops also require more than once daily dosing and may result in inadequate pupillary dilation. Early treatment is crucial in infants and young children due to the dense amblyopia that occurs with visual deprivation, which is more refractory to amblyopia treatment if treated later.

13.3 Expectations

- The expectation of pediatric cataract surgery is clearing of the visual axis to allow visual development and improvement of visual acuity.
- Intraoperatively, pediatric eyes are different from adult eyes, not only due to their smaller size and steeper corneal curvature. There is less corneal and scleral rigidity, the capsule is more elastic, and greater inflammation can occur postoperatively.[3] There is increased posterior pressure, which can result in easy shallowing of the anterior chamber during surgery. In addition, the smooth muscle tone of the iris dilator is reduced, similar to that seen in intraoperative floppy iris syndrome in adults on systemic alpha-1 antagonist medications.[4]
- The visual acuity in infants with cataracts associated with persistent fetal vasculature (PFV) may be limited by other ocular abnormalities including abnormal macular anatomy. PFV has a higher risk of complications such as hemorrhage and glaucoma, and is also commonly associated with microphthalmia, resulting in more challenging cataract surgery.
- The visual prognosis due to amblyopia and long-term monitoring and treatment is discussed with the patient's family who should understand that refractive correction will be needed postoperatively and bifocal glasses will be needed for children 2 to 3 years of age and older.

13.4 Key Principles

- The timing of surgery for congenital cataracts should be before 6 weeks of age for unilateral cataracts and before 2 months of age for bilateral cataracts,[5,6] scheduled a maximum of 2 weeks apart.
- For young children with "borderline" cataracts, once it is determined that nonsurgical treatments including pupillary dilation, correction of significant refractive error, and/or occlusion therapy are not adequately improving the visual acuity, cataract surgery is considered.

- The cataract and lens material are removed, leaving capsular support for intraocular lens (IOL) placement at the time of cataract extraction or when the child is older.
- Phacoemulsification is rarely, if ever, needed in the removal of pediatric cataracts, so the surgeon may use bimanual irrigation-aspiration handpieces or bimanual irrigation and anterior vitrectomy handpieces, which can be used for both aspiration and cutting.
- A posterior capsulotomy with anterior vitrectomy is performed during most pediatric cataract surgeries due to the rapid posterior capsule opacification that occurs in infants and young children,[7] which results in recurrence of visual deprivation, requiring additional surgical treatment.
- Anterior vitrectomy is recommended at the time of posterior capsulotomy, as the anterior hyaloid face can act as a scaffold for proliferating lens epithelial cells if only a posterior capsulorhexis is performed.[1]
- Placement of an IOL requires a larger wound, and the IOL can act as a scaffold for proliferating lens epithelial cells, which can result in recurrence of visual deprivation, even after posterior capsulotomy and anterior vitrectomy. The Infant Aphakia Treatment Study (IATS) has recommended leaving infants less than 7 months of age aphakic due to a greater frequency of adverse events and additional surgical procedures with IOL placement in this age group.[8,9] The Toddler Aphakia and Pseudophakia Study found that IOL placement is safe in children older than 6 months and younger than 2 years of age.[10] IOL implantation done later may also allow the IOL power to be chosen with better accuracy.
- Visually significant cataracts occurring in older children and teenagers, who are not at risk of developing amblyopia, are treated with implantation of an IOL with or without a posterior capsulotomy with anterior vitrectomy, depending on the patient's expected ability to tolerate laser capsulotomy, if needed.
- Following cataract extraction, the refractive error is determined and corrected with extended-wear contact lenses and/or with glasses, ideally within 2 to 3 weeks, with the understanding that the refractive error will change over time.

13.5 Indications

- In preverbal infants and toddlers with cataracts, a poor fixation behavior with a strong ocular preference, if the cataract is unilateral, and a poor red reflex through an undilated pupil are indicative of visual deprivation and warrant cataract surgery.[1]
- When the visual acuity can be reliably measured in a child and is at least in the 20/30 range in both eyes, which would allow driving in most states in the United States, or is in the 20/50 range with normal visual acuity in the fellow eye, the surgeon should have a discussion with the family regarding the balance of the potential benefits and risks of pediatric cataract surgery, as well as the timing of surgery.[11]
- Older children and teenagers who are not at risk of amblyopia are treated with cataract surgery if the vision is decreased and affecting daily activities, similar to the indications for adult cataracts.

13.6 Contraindications

There are few relative contraindications for cataract surgery in infancy and early childhood due to the dense amblyopia that occurs from visual deprivation.

- If the cataract is due to trauma with other severe ocular injuries that increase the risk of complications and limit the visual potential, cataract surgery may not be recommended.
- Cataracts with significant zonular instability due to trauma or connective tissue disorders may be best addressed by a vitreoretinal surgeon with co-management in the early postoperative period, followed by continued management of amblyopia by the pediatric ophthalmologist.
- Weighing the risks and benefits of cataract surgery in children with cataracts that appear "borderline" amblyogenic should be discussed with the patient's family, including the extensive postoperative care that is required which may be challenging for some families, so that the potentially limited visual improvement may be slightly outweighed by the risks.
- The recommendation for IOL placement depends on the age of the child, as per IATS recommendations, and also the family's ability to manage care of contact lenses, particularly in unilateral cataracts. Although implantation of an IOL is not an absolute contraindication in infants, the IATS found that young infants in whom an IOL was placed were at a significantly higher risk of requiring additional intraocular surgeries,[8] which

were generally uncomplicated but every return visit to the operating room carries risks.

- The risks of anesthesia are taken into consideration when determining the timing of surgery for children with chronic and acute diseases.

13.7 Preoperative Preparation

The assessment of a pediatric cataract includes a complete history, including the laterality, appearance, and age of onset of the cataract, as well as concerns about vision. Medical and birth history are also obtained. The examination includes an age-appropriate assessment of visual acuity, intraocular pressure, and a slit lamp examination, or at least a penlight examination of the anterior segment in infants and young children. The red reflex prior to pupillary dilation should be assessed with a retinoscope or direct ophthalmoscope to evaluate the size and location of the lens opacity relative to the visual axis. A dilated fundus examination is performed in both eyes to fully assess the lens and to examine for other ocular abnormalities that may affect visual development. Cycloplegic refraction is evaluated in both eyes to determine if a component of refractive amblyopia may be present and to aid in determining the refractive goal if IOL placement is planned for a patient with a unilateral cataract. If there is a limited view to the fundus due to the cataract, a B-scan ultrasound should be performed and a dilated fundus examination performed after the cataract is removed, either at the end of surgery while in the operating room or during a postoperative visit. Most infants and children tolerate B-scan ultrasound well, although an assessment of all quadrants of the eye may be limited. The ophthalmic examination also includes an evaluation of the ocular alignment, at least by corneal light reflex testing, as strabismus due to visual deprivation may be present. If strabismus persists or develops after cataract surgery with continued amblyopia treatment, strabismus surgery may eventually be needed. If bilateral cataracts are present, systemic causes including infectious, genetic, and metabolic diseases are considered and further evaluation recommended, usually in coordination with the patient's pediatrician. Systemic and ocular comorbidities, if present, and the morphology of the cataracts are examined to consider possible underlying etiologies of bilateral cataracts. Family history of infantile or juvenile cataracts is also obtained, in addition to examining immediate family members in the office, if possible. Lamellar

and nuclear cataracts presenting in infancy and early childhood are often familial.[1]

Cooperative children of 2 to 3 years and older may be able to undergo optical biometry in the office. If the cataract is dense or the child is not cooperative, axial length measurements with immersion A-scan ultrasound and keratometry are performed while the child is under anesthesia. The refractive goal when placing an IOL depends on the patient's age and the refraction of the fellow eye in unilateral cases. Suggested refractive goals based on age are listed in ▶ Table 13.1.[1,12] Most pediatric cataract surgeons use hydrophobic acrylic one-piece or three-piece monofocal IOLs.[13] The axial length and location of the IOL in the capsule or in the ciliary sulcus are also considered when selecting the IOL power and IOL calculation formula used. The selection of the IOL power for an intended refractive outcome is error-prone, especially in young children with smaller eyes, more shallow anterior chamber depths, changing corneal curvatures, and unpredictable axial length elongation.[1,8]

Although cyclopentolate 0.2% and phenylephrine 1% are typically used in infants for pupillary dilation, this combination may not provide adequate pupillary dilation for surgery. Cyclopentolate 1%, phenylephrine 2.5%, and mydriacyl 1% can be instilled two to three times every 5 minutes to dilate the pupils before cataract surgery. The patient is monitored while under anesthesia and in the postoperative care unit for any systemic adverse effects from the topical medications. In addition, 0.5 mL of 1:1,000 nonpreserved epinephrine per 500 mL of balanced salt solution can be added for intraocular irrigation during surgery.

An examination under anesthesia before the start of surgery may be performed to evaluate the intraocular pressure, pachymetry, gonioscopy, and precise measurements of corneal diameters if

Table 13.1 Suggested refractive goals for intraocular lens implantation in pediatric patients

Age	Refractive goal (diopters)
6–12 months	+5.00–6.00
1 year	+4.00–5.00
2 years	+4.00
3 years	+3.00
4 years	+2.00
5 years	+1.00
6–7 years	+0.50
8 years and older	Plano

unable to be reliably assessed in the office. Ocular biometry may also be performed at this time if needed. Following the examination under anesthesia, the operative eye is prepped with 5% betadine with attention to careful cleaning of the eyelashes. A fenestrated clear drape covers the patient's face and body, and a large transparent film dressing cut in half is used to completely cover the upper and lower eyelashes and position them away from the globe (▶ Fig. 13.1). The surgeon is positioned at the top of the patient's head for superior incisions which may decrease the risk of complications related to injury and endophthalmitis, and the surgical microscope is adjusted. An appropriately sized wire eyelid speculum or adjustable eyelid speculum is placed, and the eye is inspected once more under the microscope.

The instruments and medications recommended for pediatric cataract surgery are listed in ▶ Table 13.2.

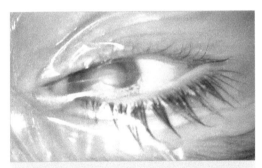

Fig. 13.1 The operative eye is draped with a clear film dressing to position the eyelashes away from the globe.

13.8 Operative Technique

13.8.1 Cataract Extraction without IOL Implantation

1. Colibri forceps are used to grasp the eye, and then a paracentesis blade is used to enter the anterior chamber at approximately 10 o'clock (▶ Fig. 13.2). A 4–0 silk traction suture can be placed around the superior rectus insertion to help position the globe during surgery.
2. Trypan blue may be used to stain the anterior capsule to better visualize the capsule for the capsulotomy.
3. Once the anterior capsule is stained, the anterior chamber is irrigated with balanced salt solution and then filled with viscoelastic.
4. A nick in the anterior capsule can be made with a cystotome needle. If the anterior capsule is smooth without a membranous plaque, a capsulorhexis can be performed using small incision forceps, such as ILM forceps, through the paracentesis wound. Alternatively, a second paracentesis wound is created at approximately 2 o'clock, 100 to 120 degrees away from the first wound, and the bimanual anterior vitrectomy handpieces are used for a vitrectorhexis (▶ Fig. 13.3). The anterior vitrector is inserted with the port initially facing down to start the anterior capsulotomy at the nick created with the cystotome (▶ Fig. 13.4a). Suggested settings for a 23-gauge anterior vitrector are a cut rate of 800 cuts per minute (cpm), maximum vacuum of 100 to 150 mmHg, and aspiration of 20 to 30 mL/minute in I/A-cut mode. A high

Table 13.2 Instruments and medications for pediatric cataract surgery

Instruments and supplies	Medications
• Appropriate size wire eyelid or adjustable eyelid speculum • Colibri fine toothed forceps • Paracentesis blade or 23-gauge MVR blade • Keratome and/or crescent blade if IOL placement is planned • Combination cohesive-dispersive viscoelastic • Cystotome needle • ILM retina forceps • 23-gauge bimanual aspiration and anterior vitrectomy handpieces • 10–0 polyglactin suture • Appropriately sized eye shield, preferably one that is clear • Eye pads • Paper tape cut with scissors or transparent film dressing	• 1:1,000 nonpreserved epinephrine added to the balanced salt solution for intraocular irrigation • Balanced salt solution on a blunt cannula • Trypan blue • Intraocular acetylcholine • Filtered air • Subconjunctival cefazoline 50 mg • Subconjunctival dexamethasone 2 mg • Prednisolone 1% • Antibiotic eye drop such as moxifloxacin • Antibiotic-steroid combination ointment • Timolol 0.5% • Atropine 1%

Abbreviation: IOL, intraocular lens.

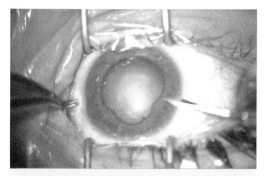

Fig. 13.2 Colibri forceps are used to stabilize the globe for the paracentesis wound. Note the small areas of iris adhesion to the anterior capsule which were dissected with viscoelastic.

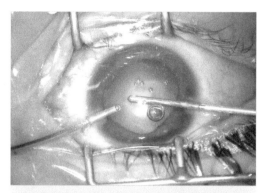

Fig. 13.3 Bimanual 23-gauge anterior vitrectomy handpieces are introduced into the eye through two paracentesis wounds approximately 120 degrees apart. The anterior capsule has been stained with Trypan blue.

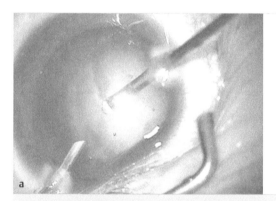

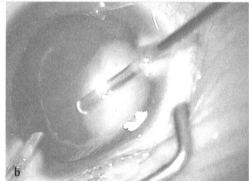

Fig. 13.4 (a) The port of the anterior vitrector initially faces down to engage the anterior capsule and then may be rotated to face up while enlarging the anterior capsulotomy. In this case, (a) a membranous plaque on the anterior capsule precluded a manual continuous capsulorhexis, and (b) a vitrectorhexis was performed.

irrigation pressure is used during surgery to help maintain the anterior chamber. An anterior chamber maintainer is helpful if the anterior chamber shallows easily during surgery. The port may then be rotated to face up (▶ Fig. 13.4b) to enlarge the capsulotomy without prematurely removing lens material to protect the posterior capsule. The anterior capsular opening should be round and approximately 5 mm, slightly smaller than the size of the dilated pupil in most patients. The bimanual anterior vitrectomy handpieces may be switched to ensure a centered and round anterior capsulotomy.

5. Next, the anterior vitrector is used to remove the lens material, primarily with aspiration. Suggested settings are maximum vacuum of 400 mmHg and aspiration of 20 to 25 mL/min,

with a cut rate of 250 cpm used intermittently for clearing the port when needed. The handpieces can be switched to completely remove peripheral cortical material with a stripping motion once the cortex is engaged. Bimanual irrigation and aspiration handpieces can also be used for removal of the cortex.

6. The anterior vitrector is then used to create a posterior capsulotomy (▶ Fig. 13.5a). Posterior capsulorhexis with a cystotome and small incision forceps has also been described. Suggested settings are to use cut-I/A mode and increase the cut rate to 1,000 cpm, and maximum vacuum of 100 to 150 mmHg. The posterior capsulotomy is enlarged to be similar in size to the anterior capsulotomy (▶ Fig. 13.5b).

7. An anterior vitrectomy is then performed to include the space under all 360 degrees of the

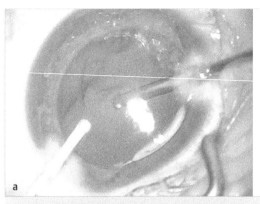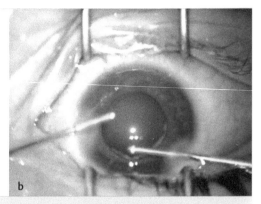

a

b

Fig. 13.5 The anterior vitrector is used to create a posterior capsulotomy once the lens material has been removed. **(a)** The port initially faces down to engage the posterior capsule, and **(b)** the size of the posterior capsulotomy is made to be similar in size to the anterior capsulotomy, slightly smaller than the dilated pupil and approximately 5 mm **(b)**. Viscoelastic is visible in panel **(a)**.

posterior capsular opening. Suggested settings are to use cut-I/A mode with a high cut rate of 1,000 to 1,500 cpm, and maximum vacuum of 100 to 150 mmHg. The vitrector is then positioned in the anterior chamber to remove any vitreous that may have migrated forward and any remaining viscoelastic.

8. Acetylcholine is then injected into the anterior chamber either on a blunt cannula or by injecting through the infusion line before the instruments are removed from the eye. The pupil will constrict and should remain round. If there is peaking of the miotic pupil due to distortion from anteriorly prolapsed vitreous, additional anterior vitrectomy is performed in the anterior chamber.

9. If the patient is to be left aphakic, the cut rate is then decreased to a very low rate with low vacuum at 100 mmHg in I/A-cut mode. With the port of the vitrector facing down over the superior peripheral iris, a surgical iridotomy is created, usually with one cut (▶ Fig. 13.6). Bleeding may occur at the iridotomy site which can usually be controlled by repressurizing the anterior chamber with irrigation.

10. The cut rate is then increased again in cut-I/A mode with the port facing up. The anterior vitrector is kept cutting as the instruments are withdrawn from the anterior chamber with the port facing up or to one side to avoid inadvertent engagement of the iris. Cellulose sponges are used to assess the wounds for vitreous, while also inspecting the pupillary margin for movement indicating the

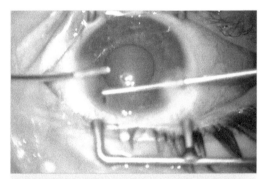

Fig. 13.6 Using a low cut rate and low maximum vacuum, the anterior vitrector is used to create a peripheral iridotomy in patients left aphakic. Mild bleeding may occur, which can usually be controlled by maintaining pressure in the anterior chamber with irrigation.

presence of vitreous to the wound, which may be manually cut first, and then additional anterior vitrectomy is performed in the anterior chamber.

11. The paracentesis wounds are closed with 10–0 polyglactin suture and rotated to bury the knot as much as possible toward the conjunctival side of the limbus. The irrigation handpiece may be kept in place while closing the first wound to help maintain the anterior chamber while placing the first suture.

12. Balanced salt solution is used to inflate the anterior chamber to a physiologic intraocular pressure by palpation. A bubble of filtered air

may be injected into the anterior chamber to prevent influx of fluid.

13. The wounds are checked again with cellulose sponges to ensure they are watertight.

14. Subconjunctival injections of cefazolin and dexamethasone are administered in the superior quadrants.

13.8.2 Cataract Extraction with IOL Implantation

There are several different approaches to pediatric cataract surgery with IOL implantation depending on whether an anterior vitrectomy is performed and the type of wound preferred by the surgeon for insertion of the IOL. Some surgeons prefer a scleral tunnel incision, while others use a corneal incision, which leaves the conjunctiva intact and through which maneuvering of instruments may be less challenging. Corneal incisions do not induce significantly greater astigmatism than scleral tunnel incisions in children.[14] Some surgeons prefer to perform the posterior capsulotomy and anterior vitrectomy after IOL placement in the capsular bag to decrease the risk of inadvertent posterior placement of the IOL, either by an anterior approach by positioning the anterior vitrector posterior to the IOL, which temporarily shifts the lens off-center and may risk injury to the capsule or zonules, or by a pars plana approach using a vitrector through a sclerostomy, which may be challenging for surgeons accustomed to anterior segment surgery. All wounds are sutured at the conclusion of surgery:

1. Steps 1 to 7 of Cataract Extraction without IOL Implantation are performed. With this method, the posterior capsulotomy and anterior vitrectomy are performed prior to IOL placement.

   a) If a scleral tunnel incision is used for IOL placement, a partial-thickness scleral tunnel is created superiorly prior to removal of the cataract. First, a 3 to 4 clock hour superior conjunctival peritomy at the limbus is created and dissected to bare sclera, followed by light cautery on the sclera for hemostasis. A partial-thickness scleral incision approximately 0.3 mm in depth is made 2.0 mm posterior to the limbus, and approximately 3 to 4 mm in length and tangential or slightly curvilinear to the limbus. A scleral tunnel is then created with a crescent blade by dissecting anteriorly to clear cornea before entering the anterior

chamber. The anterior chamber is entered with a keratome, and this incision may be used for the capsulorhexis, removal of the cataract and lens material using a coaxial irrigation-aspiration handpiece, and then for IOL insertion if posterior capsulotomy and anterior vitrectomy are not planned. Alternatively, the anterior chamber is not entered until IOL placement, and the cataract is removed using two paracentesis wounds with bimanual handpieces with or without a posterior capsulotomy and anterior vitrectomy.

2. Viscoelastic is injected into the posterior chamber to create space between the anterior and posterior capsule remnants or in the ciliary sulcus for placement of the IOL and to help keep the eye formed. An anterior chamber maintainer can also be considered at this time.

3. An appropriately sized keratome is used to enter the anterior chamber by enlarging one of the paracentesis wounds aiming for a two- or three-planed corneal incision, or through the scleral tunnel as described. A 10–0 polyglactin double-mattress suture may be loosely preplaced before the corneal wound is enlarged, with care not to cut the suture with the keratome, as a soft eye at the conclusion of surgery can be challenging to suture.

4. The selected IOL is loaded into the proper cartridge and injector. A one-piece IOL may conform better to the infant capsule,[15] although placement in the capsule can be more challenging after posterior capsulotomy. A three-piece IOL may also be placed in the ciliary sulcus with IOL folding forceps. The lens is inserted and properly positioned, ensuring that neither haptic is positioned behind the posterior capsule if a posterior capsulotomy was performed. Optic capture by prolapsing the optic posteriorly may decrease the risk of pupillary capture and posterior opacification, and stabilize lens centration but does risk posterior displacement or tilting of the IOL.[16]

5. The bimanual anterior vitrector is then re-introduced into the anterior chamber and used to remove any vitreous and remaining viscoelastic. If a corneal incision was used for IOL placement, the anterior chamber will be more difficult to maintain at this point. If a scleral tunnel incision was used, it can be closed with a double-mattress 10–0 nylon suture to better maintain the anterior chamber.

6. Acetylcholine is then instilled into the anterior chamber either on a blunt cannula or by

injecting through the infusion line before the instruments are removed from the eye. The pupil will constrict and should remain round. If there is peaking of the miotic pupil due to distortion from anteriorly prolapsed vitreous, additional anterior vitrectomy is performed.

7. The anterior vitrector is kept running and withdrawn with the port facing up or to one side to avoid inadvertent engagement of the iris. Cellulose sponges are used to evaluate the wounds for vitreous, while inspecting the pupillary margin for movement indicating the presence of vitreous to the wound, which may be manually cut first, and then additional anterior vitrectomy is performed in the anterior chamber.

8. The corneal wounds are closed with 10–0 polyglactin suture and rotated to bury the knot as much as possible toward the conjunctival side of the limbus. The irrigation handpiece may be kept in place while closing the first wound to help maintain the anterior chamber while placing the first suture. If a clear corneal incision was used for IOL placement, it may be closed with the preplaced double-mattress 10–0 polyglactin suture, in a figure 8 formation or with interrupted sutures. If a scleral tunnel incision was used and was closed with 10–0 nylon suture after IOL placement, the conjunctival peritomy is closed at the limbus with 8–0 polyglactin suture.

9. Balanced salt solution is used to inflate the anterior chamber to a physiologic intraocular pressure by palpation. A bubble of filtered air may be injected into the anterior chamber to prevent influx of fluid.

10. The wounds are checked again with cellulose sponges to ensure they are watertight.

11. Subconjunctival injections of cefazolin and dexamethasone are administered in the superior quadrants.

13.8.3 Secondary IOL Implantation

For secondary IOL placement following prior cataract surgery with posterior capsulotomy and anterior vitrectomy, the presence of capsular support for an IOL should be confirmed prior to surgery. If there is concern for poor capsular support, a sutured IOL may be needed and should be performed by a surgeon experienced with this procedure. The long-term data for sutured IOLs in children is limited; thus, extended-wear aphakic contact lenses with bifocal glasses can also be continued, as long as the patient and family tolerate this treatment. An iris claw lens placed in the anterior chamber has been developed as an alternative to a sutured IOL but is currently under investigation in the United States and not approved by the Food and Drug Administration.[17]

1. A paracentesis blade is used to enter the anterior chamber at approximately 10 o'clock and at 2 o'clock, 100 to 120 degrees apart. A 4–0 silk traction suture can be placed around the superior rectus insertion to help position the globe during surgery.

   a) If a scleral tunnel incision is to be used for IOL placement, a partial-thickness scleral tunnel is created superiorly. First, a 3 to 4 clock hour superior conjunctival peritomy at the limbus is created and dissected to bare sclera, followed by light cautery on the sclera for hemostasis. A partial-thickness scleral incision approximately 0.3 mm in depth is made 2.0 mm posterior to the limbus, and approximately 3 to 4 mm in length and tangential or slightly curvilinear to the limbus. A scleral tunnel is then created with a crescent blade by dissecting anteriorly to clear cornea before entering the anterior chamber. The anterior chamber is not entered until IOL placement following anterior vitrectomy.

2. Adhesions that may have formed between the iris and the capsule can be dissected with viscoelastic on a cannula.

3. The bimanual anterior vitrector handpieces are introduced into the anterior chamber to perform an anterior vitrectomy and to enlarge the capsulotomy to approximately 5 mm if capsular phimosis has developed. Suggested settings are to use cut-I/A mode and a high cut rate of 1,000 cpm, and maximum vacuum of 100 to 150 mmHg. The anterior vitrectomy is performed to include the space under all 360 degrees of the capsular opening. The vitrector may then be positioned in the anterior chamber to remove any vitreous that may have migrated forward.

4. If a one-piece IOL is to be implanted between the anterior and posterior capsule remnants, the capsule remnants are separated 360 degrees with viscoelastic to create space for the IOL, and remaining cortex and Soemmering's ring is carefully removed with the anterior vitrector using aspiration. If a three-piece IOL is to be implanted in the ciliary sulcus, viscoelastic is used to create space in the sulcus for the lens.

5. The surgery can then proceed with steps 3 to 11 of *Cataract Extraction with IOL Implantation* for placement of the secondary IOL.

13.9 Tips and Pearls

- During creation of the corneal wounds, the blade should slightly nick the limbal vessels for better healing and integrity of the wounds. However, the wounds should not be initiated too far posterior to the limbus to avoid ballooning of the conjunctiva during surgery. The two paracentesis wounds should be approximately 100 to 120 degrees apart for comfortable positioning of the bimanual handpieces.
- If performing a capsulorhexis with forceps, the flap of the capsule is directed nearly radially toward the center of the lens due to the elasticity of the pediatric lens capsule, rather than tangentially, as is done for an adult cataract. This direction of movement is adjusted as the capsulorhexis is advanced to achieve the desired size of the capsulotomy.
- For pediatric cataracts, the cortical material is easily stripped from the capsule without hydrodissection.
- Complete removal of the lens material is important for reducing the proliferation of lens epithelial cells and postoperative inflammation. Use of bimanual handpieces helps to thoroughly remove the lens material and also maintain the anterior chamber using smaller wounds.
- A small peripheral iridotomy is recommended for patients left aphakic to decrease the risk of pupillary block even following anterior vitrectomy.
- During IOL placement after posterior capsulotomy and anterior vitrectomy, the surgeon must be certain that both haptics are in the same plane, whether it is in the capsule or in the ciliary sulcus. More importantly, the surgeon must be certain that the haptics are not positioned behind the posterior capsular remnant before releasing the IOL:
  - If a three-piece IOL is placed in the ciliary sulcus, ensure that the leading haptic is in the sulcus first, then advance the IOL so that the optic rests in the sulcus or on the iris. Then a Kuglen hook or forceps can be used to position the optic and trailing haptic into the sulcus.
- If a three-piece IOL is used, recall that the lens should have a "2" configuration for the optic to be posteriorly vaulted. If using an IOL injector, once the leading haptic is confirmed to be in the correct position, the injector requires a small counter-clockwise rotation to ensure that the optic and trailing haptic are correctly positioned.
- Most families who will be caring for children undergoing cataract surgery and providing the postoperative care will understandably experience significant stress, especially during the early postoperative period. The family should be able to contact the surgeon without difficulty to address questions and concerns.

13.10 What to Avoid

- Unintentional injury to the iris.
- Corneal wound leak.
- An appropriately sized capsulotomy is approximately 5 mm:
  - A capsulotomy that is too small increases the risk of capsular phimosis which may be visually significant, may prevent an adequate view of the peripheral retina, and may give the eye an undesired appearance.
  - A capsulotomy that is too large may not provide adequate support for an IOL and is more difficult to visualize intraoperatively, which may impede proper positioning of the IOL.
- If a scleral tunnel incision is used for IOL placement, the scleral tunnel should be of appropriate depth:
  - A scleral tunnel that is too deep results in a scleral flap that is thick, with which intraocular maneuvering of instruments may be more difficult, and the keratome may enter the anterior chamber earlier than anticipated near the iris root, which may result in hyphema formation.
  - A scleral tunnel that is too superficial results in a scleral flap that is thin, prone to tearing, and may be more difficult to suture closed.

13.11 Complications

Early complications include intraocular hemorrhage, postoperative uveitis, endophthalmitis, elevated intraocular pressure, and the need for additional surgery, most often due to rapid proliferation of lens epithelial cells. The risk of cystoid macular edema is very low in the pediatric population.[18] Other complications include synechiae formation, iris capture at a corneal wound or pupillary capture by the IOL, IOL decentration, development of inflammatory deposits or pupillary membrane on the IOL, and retinal detachment.

A long-term complication that is monitored for the patient's lifetime is the development of glaucoma.[19] The definitive reason for the risk of glaucoma after pediatric cataract surgery remains unclear and does not appear to be related to IOL placement,[1] while microphthalmia with microcornea and younger age in infancy at the time of surgery appear to be risk factors for the development of glaucoma after pediatric cataract surgery.[20]

If an IOL was placed, development of visual axis or posterior capsule opacification is monitored and treated if there is recurrence of visual deprivation. Corneal scarring at the corneal wounds may be visible but usually fade over time. Amblyopia that develops due to visual deprivation preoperatively may not respond fully, even with compliant amblyopia treatment after surgery. There is also a risk of corneal ulcer with the use of extended-wear contact lenses used for aphakia.

13.12 Postoperative Care

At the conclusion of pediatric cataract surgery, the eye is patched and shielded after instillation of prednisolone 1%, an antibiotic eye drop such as moxifloxacin, and an antibiotic-corticosteroid combination ointment. Atropine 0.5 to 1% and timolol 0.5% may also be instilled, as well as an additional drop of 5% betadine. The shield may be secured with paper tape or with transparent film dressings. The patch is kept in place overnight and removed by the physician on postoperative day 1. In extenuating circumstances, bilateral cataract surgery may be performed using completely separate surgical packs with different lot numbers. The first eye is patched and shielded during the second eye surgery. The second eye is then patched and shielded, and the first eye is shielded after instillation of a second set of topical antibiotic and steroid at the conclusion of the bilateral surgery. The eye drop regimen is started on postoperative day 1 as follows: prednisolone 1% six times daily or more often, depending on the concern for postoperative inflammation, moxifloxacin four times daily, and antibiotic-corticosteroid ointment nightly. The family is advised to shake the prednisolone bottle well before every use. If the intraocular pressure is elevated, the timolol that was instilled at the conclusion of surgery is also started. Infants and young children should

not receive alpha-2 adrenergic agonists, such as brimonidine, due to the risk of central nervous system effects including somnolence and apnea. A clear shield is used to protect the eye at all times for the first 1 to 2 weeks after surgery. If the patient wears glasses, they may be worn during the day in place of the shield, with the shield used while sleeping and with the understanding that the glasses prescription will need to be updated. Moxifloxacin and the antibiotic-corticosteroid ointment is continued for 1 to 2 weeks postoperatively, and prednisolone is tapered over approximately 4 to 6 weeks, depending on the degree of postoperative intraocular inflammation. Postoperative appointments are then scheduled at 1 week, 2 to 4 weeks, 1 to 3 months, and 6 months, with additional visits if there are any concerns or complications.

Strict return precautions are discussed with the family, particularly symptoms that may signify early endophthalmitis. Pain, worsening redness of the eye, discharge, worsening eyelid edema and erythema, decreased vision, or other concerns should be addressed and evaluated promptly.

If a visual axis or posterior capsule opacification develops in a patient who does not tolerate laser treatment in the office, the treatment can be performed under general anesthesia at some surgical centers, if the laser can be transported to the operating room and the patient can be safely positioned in the laser, usually requiring more than one person for assistance. Alternatively, a pars plana approach to clear the visual axis opacification with vitrectomy, performed by a vitreoretinal surgeon, can be done if laser treatment is not possible or is ultimately unable to achieve a satisfactory result. The response of visual axis opacification to laser treatment in pediatric patients differs from laser capsulotomy in adults. In children, laser treatment often results in small, irregular openings within the opacification, although the openings may be adequate to resolve visual deprivation. In addition, laser treatment may require repeat treatments, as the lens epithelial cells continue to reproliferate over the IOL.

Amblyopia treatment continues in the postoperative period and depends on whether the cataract was unilateral or bilateral, on the patient's age, and whether the patient was left aphakic or an IOL was placed. Refractive correction is provided with extended-wear contact

Table 13.3 Optimizing refraction correction for amblyopia treatment in various scenarios after pediatric cataract surgery. Occlusion therapy is also often indicated, especially in unilateral cases

| Laterality | Lens status | |
	Aphakia	*Pseudophakia*
Unilateral	• Until 2 to 3 years of age, an extended-wear contact lens is overplussed by 2 to 3 diopters to provide intermediate to near correction • After 2 to 3 years of age, an extended-wear contact lens that is not overplussed and a bifocal lens in glasses for the aphakic eye are used, as long as the patient tolerates the contact lens or until an IOL is implanted • Glasses are not a suitable option due to aniseikonia that occurs due to the large degree of anisometropia	• Until 2 to 3 years of age, refractive correction with glasses may be slightly overplussed for the pseudophakic eye only • After 2 to 3 years of age, a bifocal lens for the pseudophakic eye may be added without overplussing
Bilateral	• Until 2 to 3 years of age, either glasses or extended-wear contact lenses that are overplussed by 2 to 3 diopters to provide intermediate to near correction • Extended-wear contact lenses may be preferred for amblyopia treatment due to the aberrations that occur with very high hyperopic correction in glasses, which could negatively impact amblyopia treatment; however, some families strongly prefer treatment with glasses due to the stress of placing and caring for contact lenses in a young child • Starting at 2 to 3 years of age, patients may wear extended-wear contact lenses without overplussing and bifocal glasses for as long as the patient tolerates the contact lenses or until IOLs are implanted • Bifocal lenses in aphakic glasses may be challenging to use due to the lens thickness and additional aberrations, and secondary IOL placement may be considered once bifocal glasses are needed	• Until 2 to 3 years of age, refractive correction with glasses overplussed by 2 to 3 diopters • After 2 to 3 years of age, a bifocal is added and the prescription is no longer overplussed

Abbreviation: IOL, intraocular lens.

lenses and/or with glasses ideally within 2 to 3 weeks after surgery. Occlusion therapy for unilateral cataracts and for bilateral cataracts with asymmetric visual development is also started within 2 to 3 weeks after surgery and continued until maximal visual acuity improvement is achieved and maintained. Extended-wear silicone elastomer contact lenses are available for infants in one diameter (11.3 mm), three base curves (7.5, 7.7, 7.9), and a range in power from +23.00 diopters to +32.00 diopters in 3.00 diopter increments. With the correct power based on retinoscopy, a base curve of 7.5 can be chosen empirically for most infants, and a base curve of 7.7 can be used for children 2 to 3 years of age. Ideally, the lenses are removed nightly and stored, but for some children, removal every 2 to 4 weeks may best suit the family. Some surgeons place the first contact lens, usually +29 or +32, at the conclusion of surgery and no postoperative ointment is used. Suggestions for optimizing the refractive correction in various scenarios are outlined in ▶ Table 13.3.

References

[1] Drummond GT, Hinz BJ. Management of monocular cataract with long-term dilation in children. Can J Ophthalmol. 1994; 29(5):227–230

[2] Pooniya V, Pandey N. Systemic toxicity of topical cyclopentolate eyedrops in a child. Eye (Lond). 2012; 26(10):1391–1392

[3] Medsinge A, Nischal KK. Pediatric cataract: challenges and future directions. Clin Ophthalmol. 2015; 9:77–90

[4] Wilson ME, Saunders RA, Trivedi RH, Eds. Pediatric Ophthalmology: Current Thought and a Practical Guide. Leipzig, Germany: Springer; 2009

[5] Birch EE, Stager DR. The critical period for surgical treatment of dense congenital unilateral cataract. Invest Ophthalmol Vis Sci. 1996; 37(8):1532–1538

[6] Birch EE, Cheng C, Stager DR, Jr, Weakley DR, Jr, Stager DR, Sr. The critical period for surgical treatment of dense congenital bilateral cataracts. J AAPOS. 2009; 13(1):67–71

[7] Jensen AA, Basti S, Greenwald MJ, Mets MB. When may the posterior capsule be preserved in pediatric intraocular lens surgery? Ophthalmology. 2002; 109(2):324–327, discussion 328

[8] Lambert SR, Lynn MJ, Hartmann EE, et al. Infant Aphakia Treatment Study Group. Comparison of contact lens and intraocular lens correction of monocular aphakia during infancy: a randomized clinical trial of HOTV optotype acuity at age 4.5 years and clinical findings at age 5 years. JAMA Ophthalmol. 2014; 132(6):676–682

[9] Lambert SR, Aakalu VK, Hutchinson AK, et al. Intraocular lens implantation during early childhood: a report by the American Academy of Ophthalmology. Ophthalmology. 2019; 126(10): 1454–1461

[10] Bothun ED, Wilson ME, Traboulsi EI, et al. Toddler Aphakia and Pseudophakia Study Group (TAPS). Outcomes of unilateral cataracts in infants and toddlers 7 to 24 months of age: Toddler Aphakia and Pseudophakia Study (TAPS). Ophthalmology. 2019; 126(8):1189–1195

[11] Wilson ME. Pediatric Cataracts: Overview. AAO Knights Templar Eye Foundation Pediatric Ophthalmology Education Center. https://www.aao.org/disease-review/pediatric-cataracts-overview. Published 2015. Accessed February 13, 2020

[12] Indaram M, VanderVeen DK. Postoperative refractive errors following pediatric cataract extraction with intraocular lens implantation. Semin Ophthalmol. 2018; 33(1): 51–58

[13] Wilson ME, Jr, Trivedi RH, Buckley EG, et al. ASCRS white paper. Hydrophobic acrylic intraocular lenses in children. J Cataract Refract Surg. 2007; 33(11):1966–1973

[14] Bar-Sela SM, Spierer A. Astigmatism outcomes of scleral tunnel and clear corneal incisions for congenital cataract surgery. Eye (Lond). 2006; 20(9):1044–1048

[15] Wilson ME, Jr, Englert JA, Greenwald MJ. In-the-bag secondary intraocular lens implantation in children. J AAPOS. 1999; 3(6): 350–355

[16] Xie YB, Ren MY, Wang Q, Wang LH. Intraocular lens optic capture in pediatric cataract surgery. Int J Ophthalmol. 2018; 11(8):1403–1410

[17] Gawdat GI, Taher SG, Salama MM, Ali AA. Evaluation of Artisan aphakic intraocular lens in cases of pediatric aphakia with insufficient capsular support. J AAPOS. 2015; 19(3):242–246

[18] Whitman MC, Vanderveen DK. Complications of pediatric cataract surgery. Semin Ophthalmol. 2014; 29(5–6):414–420

[19] Chen TC, Walton DS, Bhatia LS. Aphakic glaucoma after congenital cataract surgery. Arch Ophthalmol. 2004; 122(12): 1819–1825

[20] Bothun ED, Wilson ME, Vanderveen DK, et al. Outcomes of bilateral cataracts removed in infants 1 to 7 months of age using the toddler aphakia and pseudophakia treatment study registry. Ophthalmology. 2020; 127(4):501–510

14 Corneal Collagen Cross-Linking for Keratoconus

Maanasa Indaram

Summary

Keratoconus is a bilateral corneal ectatic disorder characterized by progressive thinning and steepening of the cornea. This results in high amounts of irregular astigmatism and can progress to scarring, hydrops, and perforation—three outcomes requiring corneal transplantation for visual rehabilitation. Typically, the onset of keratoconus is at puberty, and it can progress until the fourth decade of life. However, there are several reports of keratoconus presenting at even younger ages. Patients diagnosed at younger ages have a significantly higher risk and pace of keratoconus progression, lending to a seven-fold higher risk of requiring corneal transplantation compared to adults. Although optical symptoms may be addressed with refractive correction, corneal collagen cross-linking (CXL) is the only definitive intervention to prevent disease progression. This chapter reviews CXL using the Dresden protocol, currently the only protocol approved by the United States Federal Drug Administration (FDA) for the treatment of keratoconus.

Keywords: keratoconus, cross-linking, riboflavin, UVA light, tomography, topography

14.1 Goals

- Stop or slow the progression of keratoconus in the long term (at least 10 years as per prior studies) by strengthening and stabilizing the collagen fibers in the cornea.[1]
- Stabilize or improve both uncorrected and corrected distance visual acuity measurements by postoperative year 1.[2,3]
- Stabilize or decrease steep keratometry values by postoperative year 1.[2,3]
- Visualize a "demarcation line" in the posterior stroma on anterior segment optical coherence tomography (AS-OCT), which is indicative of the depth of the collagen cross-linking treatment into the stroma.[4]
- Ultimately prevent vision loss and/or the need for corneal transplantation from severe progression of keratoconus.

14.2 Advantages

Corneal collagen cross-linking (CXL) stabilizes collagen fibers in the cornea to stop or slow the progression of keratoconus, thereby preventing the development of high degrees of irregular astigmatism that occurs without treatment, which can become progressively difficult to treat with specially fitted contact lenses, and decreasing the risk of serious vision-threatening complications including hydrops, severe scarring, and corneal perforation, which can place the patient at risk of needing corneal transplantation.

14.3 Expectations

- Stop or slow the progression of keratoconus for at least 10 years following treatment.
- Ocular pain in the first postoperative week while the corneal epithelial defect heals.
- Uncomplicated healing of the induced corneal epithelial defect without infection or scarring.
- Corneal haze and edema in the first postoperative month which then resolves.
- Decreased vision for up to 1 month postoperatively which then recovers to the preoperative baseline.
- Improvement of uncorrected and/or corrected visual acuity in some patients by postoperative month 6.
- As per prior long-term data, 20% of patients, especially those who are under 12 years at the time of their diagnosis, may require repeat CXL within 10 years following initial treatment due to progression, and 4% of patients may require corneal transplantation due to severe progression.[2]

14.4 Key Principles

- CXL utilizes riboflavin, a photosensitizer, with ultraviolet A (UVA) light to strengthen collagen bonds within the corneal stroma, thereby accelerating the normal process of age-related cross-linking that occurs over an individual's lifetime.[3]
- When cross-linked, the collagen fibrils of the cornea are stiffened and therefore less likely to stretch and thin the cornea.[5]

- With proper surgical technique, maximum treatment efficacy can be achieved while minimizing long-term risks, such as infectious keratitis, persistent corneal haze, or corneal scarring.

14.5 Indications

As per FDA guidelines, the following are the indications and inclusion criteria for corneal cross-linking. In clinical practice, many surgeons have a more liberal approach (especially for age) in determining candidates for CXL:[3]

- Age 14 years or older.
- Corneal topography pattern consistent with keratoconus, namely a pattern of inferior corneal steepening.
- Steep keratometry value of 47 diopters or more.
- Inferior-to-superior ratio of greater than 1.5 on corneal topography.
- Corrected distance visual acuity worse than 20/20 in the treatment eye.
- Corneal thickness greater than or equal to 300 microns.
- Evidence of keratoconus progression over a 24-month period, including an increase in the steepest keratometry measurement of 1 diopter or more, an increase in cylindrical refractive error by manifest refraction of 1 diopter or more, or an increase in manifest refraction spherical equivalent of 0.5 diopters or more.

14.6 Contraindications

- Prior history of corneal surgery, excluding prior CXL.
- Corneal pathology that could impede epithelial wound healing, such as chemical injury, neurotrophic keratopathy, or limbal stem cell disease.
- Prior history of herpetic keratitis, as CXL can cause disease re-activation.
- Severe corneal scarring or opacification.
- Severe dry eye disease.

14.7 Preoperative Preparation

- Preoperatively, a careful history is obtained and slit-lamp examination is performed to evaluate for any of the contraindications listed above.
- Placido-based corneal topography or, if available, Scheimpflug corneal tomography is obtained to document the presence of progressive keratoconus.

- A baseline AS-OCT scan is obtained for comparison with the postoperative scan.
- During the preoperative evaluation, the surgeon, the patient, and the patient's family determine if the procedure can be undertaken under topical anesthesia in a clinic-based setting or if the patient requires general anesthesia in the operating room due to concerns about patient cooperation.
- The surgeon should have a detailed preoperative discussion with the patient and the patient's family outlining the goals of treatment, namely, halting keratoconus progression. Care should be taken to ensure the patient understands that CXL does not reverse the pre-existing changes caused by keratoconus and that it is not a refractive procedure that will eliminate the need for refractive correction.

14.8 Operative Technique

14.8.1 Anesthesia and Preparation

1. For patients undergoing the procedure under topical anesthesia in the clinic, several drops of tetracaine 0.5% are instilled into the operative eye. Patients requiring general anesthesia are placed under anesthesia in the operating room.
2. Once the appropriate anesthesia is achieved, the operative eye receives one drop each of ketorolac tromethamine 0.5% and moxifloxacin 0.5% eye drops.
3. The eye is then prepped and draped in the usual sterile manner using 5% betadine ophthalmic solution.

14.8.2 Alcohol-Assisted Corneal Epithelium Removal

1. An 8 to 9 mm circular corneal epithelial well is held on the central cornea with even pressure.
2. Into the well, several drops of ethanol diluted to 20% using sterile water are instilled onto the corneal surface (▶ Fig. 14.1). The well is held in place with the ethanol over the cornea for 30 seconds, taking care not to lift any side of it and displacing the ethanol off the central cornea.
3. After 30 seconds, a cellulose sponge is used to completely wick the ethanol from the well. Then, balanced salt solution is used to gently rinse the cornea and conjunctiva of any remaining ethanol.
4. A micro-hoe is used to gently lift the epithelial edge.

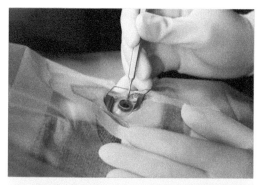

Fig. 14.1 Several drops of ethanol diluted to 20% using sterile water are instilled onto the corneal surface in an 8 to 9 mm circular corneal epithelial well held on the central cornea with even pressure.

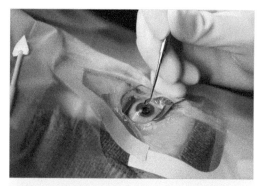

Fig. 14.2 A blunt spatula is used to remove the epithelium off the central 8 to 9 mm cornea after ethanol treatment.

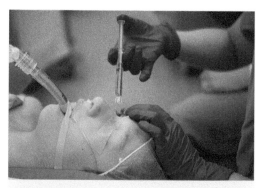

Fig. 14.3 Riboflavin is administered topically over the cornea, one drop every 2 minutes for 30 minutes.

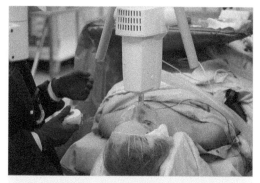

Fig. 14.4 The 8 to 9 mm of central cornea denuded of epithelium is aligned and exposed to UVA light (365 nm) for 30 minutes at an irradiance of 3.0 mW/cm².

5. Using this epithelial edge, a blunt spatula is used to peel the epithelium off the central 8 to 9 mm cornea (▶ Fig. 14.2).

14.8.3 Induction with Riboflavin

1. Riboflavin (0.1% in 20% dextran T500 solution) is administered topically over the cornea (▶ Fig. 14.3), one drop every 2 minutes for 30 minutes.
2. At the end of this conditioning period, the absorption of riboflavin through the corneal stroma is confirmed by visualizing yellow flare in the anterior chamber by portable slit-lamp examination. If this yellow flare is not visualized, the same riboflavin eye drops are administered one drop every 10 seconds for 2 minutes, after which a portable slit-lamp examination is repeated to visualize yellow flare in the anterior

chamber. This is repeated until the yellow flare is visualized.

3. Ultrasound pachymetry is performed to measure the central corneal thickness and ensure it is greater than 400 microns. If the cornea is thinner than 400 microns, hypotonic riboflavin (0.1% riboflavin without dextran) is administered one drop every 10 seconds for 2-minute sessions until a corneal thickness of at least 400 microns is achieved.

14.8.4 Treatment with Ultraviolet A (UVA) Light

1. Using the KXL® system by Avedro, which is currently the only CXL system approved by the FDA, the 8 to 9 mm of central cornea denuded of epithelium is aligned and exposed to UVA light (365 nm) for 30 minutes at an irradiance of 3.0 mW/cm² (▶ Fig. 14.4).

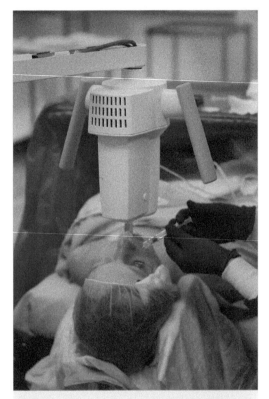

Fig. 14.5 During the period of ultraviolet A (UVA) irradiance, riboflavin eye drops are again administered topically over the cornea, one drop every 2 minutes for 30 minutes.

2. During this period of irradiance, riboflavin eye drops are again administered topically over the cornea (▶ Fig. 14.5), one drop every 2 minutes for 30 minutes.
3. At the conclusion of treatment, the cornea is rinsed thoroughly with balanced salt solution (BSS), followed by one drop each of ketorolac tromethamine 0.5%, moxifloxacin 0.5%, and prednisolone acetate 1% eye drops.
4. A bandage contact lens is then placed over the operative eye for comfort and the eye is shielded.

14.9 Tips and Pearls

- If there is a concern that the patient will be unable to tolerate the procedure while awake with topical anesthesia, including young children or patients with developmental delay, general anesthesia is recommended.
- Due to strong intracellular adhesions in young patients, removal of the central corneal

epithelium after ethanol treatment should be performed as quickly as possible to minimize any trauma to the corneal stroma caused by epithelium that re-adheres to the anterior stroma.
- Because 0.1% riboflavin eye drops in 20% dextran solution is a hypertonic and more viscous solution, it may result in some deturgescence of the cornea. For corneas that are less than 450 microns thick, of which approximately 50 microns will be removed with the epithelium, it is recommended that hypotonic riboflavin solution without dextran be used for the induction process. Note that the dextran-containing riboflavin solution was used in the clinical trial that resulted in FDA approval.
- In patients for whom bandage contact lens removal in the clinic is unlikely to be practical at the first postoperative visit, a bandage contact lens should not be placed. As an alternative for pain management due to the corneal epithelial defect, the operative eye may be patched for 3 days postoperatively.
- The procedure is almost always performed on one eye at a time to mitigate potential risks. Rarely, the procedure may be performed bilaterally on the same day. For this scenario, the central corneal epithelium is removed from both eyes at the start of the procedure. The first eye then undergoes induction with riboflavin, and the second eye is closed. While the first eye is treated with UVA light, induction of the second eye with riboflavin can occur simultaneously. Then, a bandage contact lens is placed on the first eye and the second eye undergoes treatment with UVA light.

14.10 Complications

- Persistent corneal haze beyond 1 month postoperatively.
- Infectious keratitis.
- Sterile corneal infiltrates.
- Corneal scarring.
- Limbal stem cell damage.
- Endothelial cell damage.
- Disease progression or unresponsiveness to treatment.

14.11 What to Avoid

- Complete corneal epithelial removal (i.e., limbus to limbus) or treatment of the corneal limbus with UVA light, as this may damage the limbal stem cells.

- Proceeding with UVA treatment even though yellow flare in the anterior chamber is not established, which could result in incomplete cross-linking through the corneal stroma.
- Proceeding with UVA treatment even though the corneal thickness is measured to be less than 400 microns, which could result in endothelial cell damage.

14.12 Postoperative Care and Precautions

- The patient is instructed to maintain the bandage contact lens in place through postoperative week 1, after which it is removed in the office. This ensures that the patient has adequate pain control while the cornea is re-epithelializing.
- The patient is instructed to use ketorolac tromethamine 0.5%, moxifloxacin 0.5%, and prednisolone acetate 1% eye drops four times daily for the first postoperative week, after which the ketorolac and moxifloxacin eye drops are discontinued and the prednisolone acetate eye drops are tapered over a total 4-week course.

- The patient is instructed to wear a protective eye shield while sleeping for the first postoperative week and to wear sunglasses when exposed to any sunlight, both indoors and outdoors, for 1 month postoperatively.
- Most importantly, the patient is instructed to avoid any eye rubbing during the postoperative period as this could impede wound healing and/or could result in keratoconus progression.

References

[1] Barbisan PRT, Pinto RDP, Gusmão CC, de Castro RS, Arieta CEL. Corneal collagen cross-linking in young patients for progressive keratoconus. Cornea. 2020; 39(2):186–191

[2] Mazzotta C, Traversi C, Baiocchi S, et al. Corneal collagen cross-linking with riboflavin and ultraviolet A light for pediatric keratoconus: ten-year results. Cornea. 2018; 37(5):560–566

[3] Hersh PS, Stulting RD, Muller D, Durrie DS, Rajpal RK, United States Crosslinking Study Group. United States multicenter clinical trial of corneal collagen crosslinking for keratoconus treatment. Ophthalmology. 2017; 124(9):1259–1270

[4] Spadea L, Tonti E, Vingolo EM. Corneal stromal demarcation line after collagen cross-linking in corneal ectatic diseases: a review of the literature. Clin Ophthalmol. 2016; 10:1803–1810

[5] Wollensak G, Spoerl E, Seiler T. Riboflavin/ultraviolet-a-induced collagen crosslinking for the treatment of keratoconus. Am J Ophthalmol. 2003; 135(5):620–627

Section IV

Pediatric Glaucoma Procedures

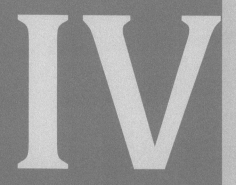

15 Goniotomy

Helen H. Yeung

Summary

Goniotomy is unique among glaucoma procedures by restoring or improving the function of the filtration angle. It is often considered to be the best initial glaucoma surgery in appropriately selected patients.

Keywords: infantile glaucoma, childhood glaucoma, goniotomy

15.1 Goals

- Lower the intraocular pressure (IOP).
- Decrease glaucoma medication usage.
- Potentially cure certain types of childhood primary and secondary glaucoma.

15.2 Advantages

- Minimally invasive procedure.
- Preserves the conjunctiva and sclera for filtration surgery if needed.

15.3 Expectations

- Results of goniotomy are variable and depend greatly on the severity of the congenital or acquired filtration angle abnormality.
- Excellent results can be expected for patients with infantile primary congenital glaucoma (PCG) and secondary glaucoma due to uveitis, while less successful results are seen in patients with Sturge-Weber syndrome and newborn PCG (patients presenting with glaucoma between birth to 1 month of age).

15.4 Key Principles

Goniotomy is done to improve filtration angle function (▶ Fig. 15.1) and can be followed by any other alternative glaucoma procedures if needed.

15.5 Indications

- The clinical indications depend on the accurate diagnostic classification of the glaucoma which determines whether the patient is a favorable candidate to benefit from goniotomy (▶ Table 15.1).
- The decision to perform a goniotomy is multifactorial and should be determined based on the experience of the surgeon and availability of appropriate surgical instruments and equipment, as well as the corneal clarity, gonioscopic findings, and history of prior glaucoma surgery.

15.6 Contraindications

- An inadequate view of the filtration angle.
- Although goniotomy is not as effective in some types of childhood glaucoma, treatment with

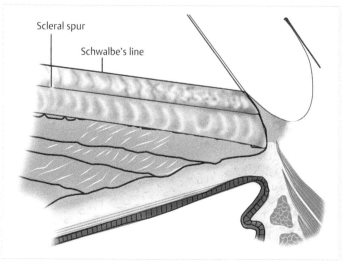

Fig. 15.1 Gonioscopic appearance of a typical filtration angle in primary congenital glaucoma.

Scleral spur

Schwalbe's line

Table 15.1 Favorable versus unfavorable types of childhood glaucoma for goniotomy

Favorable	Unfavorable
• Infantile primary congenital glaucoma	• Newborn primary congenital glaucoma
• Late-recognized primary congenital glaucoma	• Sturge-Weber syndrome
• Steroid-induced glaucoma	• Synechial angle-closure glaucoma
• Open-angle uveitic glaucoma	• Late aniridic glaucoma
• Early infantile aphakic glaucoma	• Iridocorneal endothelial syndrome
• Iridogoniodysgenesis	• Traumatic angle recession
• Prophylaxis for aniridic glaucoma	• Congenital iris ectropion syndrome

Table 15.2 Goniotomy instruments and supplies

Instruments	Supplies
• Tonometer	• Apraclonidine 0.5%
• Calipers	• Balanced salt solution
• Pediatric eyelid speculum	• 30-gauge irrigation needle or cannula
• Direct viewing gonioscopy lens	• Epinephrine 1:16,000 in a 3 mL syringe
• Surgical microscope or loupes with an illumination source	• 70% isopropyl alcohol
	• 10–0 polyglactin suture
• Locking toothed forceps such as Elschnig-O'Connor locking fixation forceps	• Antibiotic eyedrop or ointment such as bacitracin/polymyxin
• Operating gonioscopy lens of appropriate size	• Prednisolone acetate 1%
• Goniotomy knife or 25-gauge needle	
• Fine tying forceps	
• External irrigation cannula	
• #15 blade	

goniotomy may still temporarily improve the intraocular pressure in these patients until a more definitive glaucoma surgery (usually trabeculectomy or tube shunt placement) is eventually needed.

15.7 Preoperative Preparation

- It is essential that the required instruments and equipment are readily available for an uninterrupted presurgical examination under anesthesia and successful goniotomy (▶ Table 15.2).
- Topical glaucoma medications are discontinued 48 hours prior to surgery. If oral acetazolamide is being taken, it is discontinued 12 hours prior to surgery.
- Topical antibiotic ophthalmic ointment such as bacitracin/polymyxin or bacitracin is administered to both eyes at bedtime the night before surgery.[1]

15.8 Operative Technique

15.8.1 Examination Under Anesthesia

1. Once the patient is under anesthesia, tonometry, corneal diameter measurements, gonioscopy, inspection of the cornea and irides with portable slit-lamp examination, and fundoscopy are performed first.
2. During gonioscopy, the quality of the view to the angle is appraised, and the trabecular meshwork is studied to determine the site of the planned surgery.

3. Minimal apraclonidine 0.5% may be administered on a microsurgical sponge to the limbal region where the goniotomy will be performed to lessen the postoperative reflux of blood during the immediate period of hypotony that can be expected before reformation of the anterior chamber.

15.8.2 Goniotomy Procedure

1. After preparation of the surgical field in the usual sterile fashion, the eyelashes are secured with sterile tape to prevent contact with the needle or knife and to facilitate unimpeded entry through the cornea.
2. The surgeon is positioned to face the angle where surgery will be performed and may be seated if using a surgical microscope or may stand if using loupes. Initial surgery is typically done in the nasal angle, so that the surgeon is positioned temporal to the operative eye.
3. The plane of the iris is rotated away from the surgeon by positioning of the eye and patient's head.
4. Locking toothed forceps are placed at the vertical rectus muscle insertions to avoid distortion of the cornea and to facilitate entry of the goniotomy instrument through a clear corneal incision at the limbus.

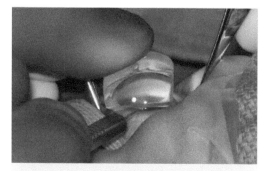

Fig. 15.2 Direct visualization of the filtration angle using an operating goniotomy lens.

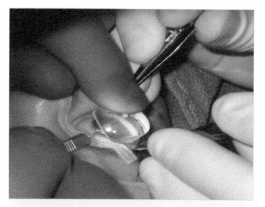

Fig. 15.3 Unimpeded entry of the goniotomy instrument away from the operating lens avoids dislodging and elevating the lens during the procedure.

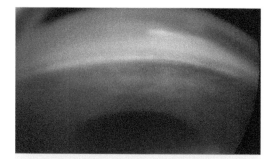

Fig. 15.4 The goniotomy knife is used in the mid-to-posterior trabecular meshwork followed by a circumferential incision for approximately 5 clock hours.

5. The procedure is done under direct observation of the angle using an operating goniotomy lens (▶ Fig. 15.2). The size of the operating lens is selected to permit comfortable, unimpeded entry of the goniotomy instrument away from the operating lens to avoid dislodging and elevating the lens during the procedure (▶ Fig. 15.3).

6. Loupes with an illumination source or the operating microscope is adjusted to provide an optimum view of the angle.

7. The goniotomy instrument is directed to enter through the cornea anterior to the limbus to allow horizontal movement of the instrument parallel to the iris.

8. Passage of the goniotomy knife across the anterior chamber is visually monitored, and its tip engaged into the mid-to-posterior trabecular meshwork followed by a circumferential incision for approximately 5 clock hours (▶ Fig. 15.4).

9. The goniotomy knife is then removed, promptly followed by deepening of the anterior chamber with balanced salt solution.

10. Typically, no additional anterior chamber irrigation is performed to remove residual refluxed blood.

11. If the reflux of blood appears excessive on inspection, approximately 0.2 mL of epinephrine 1:16,000 can be irrigated into the anterior chamber.

12. If the corneal incision appears to be leaking and the anterior chamber is not maintained, the wound is closed with a 10–0 polyglactin suture.

13. At the end of the procedure, a topical antibiotic drop, prednisolone acetate 1%, apraclonidine 0.5%, and an antibiotic ointment are instilled.[2]

15.9 Tips and Pearls

- It is important to rule out nasolacrimal duct obstruction, which is a much more common cause of tearing in infants than childhood glaucoma.
- If significant corneal epithelial edema is present, such that the view is obstructed, the epithelium can be removed by instilling 70% isopropyl alcohol to the cornea and then gently removing the epithelium with a #15 blade. Then, balanced salt solution is used to gently rinse the cornea and conjunctiva of any remaining alcohol.
- Approximately 5 days prior to surgery, an attempt can be made to clear corneal stromal edema by lowering the IOP with oral acetazolamide 10 to 15 mg/kg/day in divided doses twice to three times daily.
- When the tip of the goniotomy knife is at the optimum depth within the trabecular tissue, there

is no perceptible tactile sensation of cutting of the trabecular tissue; however, if there is a grating sensation, the position of the goniotomy knife is too deep.

- Preparation for an external trabeculotomy is always advisable when planning for a goniotomy procedure.

15.10 What to Avoid

- Inadequate view of the filtration angle determined by intraoperative gonioscopy, as this is a contraindication for goniotomy.

15.11 Complications

- Injury to any of the anterior segment structures.
- Creation of a cyclodialysis cleft.

15.12 Postoperative Care

- A topical corticosteroid is given twice daily for 1 week.

- If a corneal suture is placed, a topical antibiotic ointment is instilled once daily as long as the suture is present.
- Head of bed elevation immediately after surgery and in the postanesthesia care unit (PACU) and continued for 1 week postoperatively to decrease the risk of complications from hyphema formation.
- Hyphemas can worsen and enlarge in the presence of hypotony and must be monitored closely.
- If the hyphema worsens and is felt to be responsible for IOP elevation, an anterior chamber washout is recommended.

15.13 Acknowledgment

Special thanks to David S. Walton, MD, for his guidance during the preparation of this chapter.

References

[1] Grajewski AL, Bitrian E, Papadopoulos M, Freedman SF. Surgical Management of Childhood Glaucoma. Cham, Switzerland: Springer; 2018:49–55

[2] Thomas JV, Belcher CD, Simmons RJ. Glaucoma Surgery. St. Louis, MO: Mosby Year Book; 1992:107–121

16 Trabeculotomy

Helen H. Yeung

Summary

Trabeculotomy is another form of angle surgery that can be considered for the treatment of children with infantile glaucoma.

Keywords: infantile glaucoma, trabeculotomy

16.1 Goals

- Lower the intraocular pressure (IOP).
- Decrease glaucoma medication usage.

16.2 Advantages

Although goniotomy is the preferred first-line procedure for primary infantile glaucoma, trabeculotomy is an alternative method of treatment when there is poor visibility of the angle.

16.3 Expectations

- The results of trabeculotomy depend on patient selection, similar to goniotomy.
- Best results are achieved with infantile primary congenital glaucoma.
- A small hyphema is usually present at the conclusion of the procedure and may persist for 1 to 2 days.

16.4 Key Principles

- Trabeculotomy is considered when there is poor visibility of the angle, impeding the ability to perform goniotomy.

16.5 Indications

- Trabeculotomy may be used for the same types of glaucoma for which goniotomy is indicated.
- The degree of difficulty of a trabeculotomy is not increased in the presence of corneal clouding to the same extent as a goniotomy.
- Trabeculotomy is reserved for those cases when corneal clouding or opacification results in an inadequate view for a goniotomy.

16.6 Preoperative Preparation

Ensure that the required instruments and equipment are readily available for an uninterrupted presurgical examination under anesthesia and successful trabeculotomy (▶ Table 16.1). Once the patient is under anesthesia, tonometry, corneal diameter measurements, gonioscopy, inspection of the cornea and irides with portable slit-lamp examination, and fundoscopy are performed first.

16.7 Operative Technique

1. The procedure is performed superotemporally or superonasally to avoid areas that may be needed for a trabeculectomy in the future.
2. A conjunctival peritomy is created with two relaxing incisions and dissected down to bare sclera. This is followed by the creation of a 3.5-mm triangular limbus-based scleral flap (▶ Fig. 16.1) using a #57 Beaver blade or a scarifier.
3. Dissection of this flap is extended anteriorly toward the cornea until the darker limbal tissue is easily visualized at a depth of approximately one half of the scleral thickness.
4. An anterior chamber paracentesis wound is created with a paracentesis blade, either superonasally or superotemporally, depending on patient and surgeon positioning.
5. The paracentesis allows entry of a short, 30-gauge cannula for re-formation of the anterior chamber and should be of adequate length to be self-sealing.

Table 16.1 Trabeculotomy instruments and supplies

Instruments	Supplies
• Surgical microscope	• Balanced salt solution
• Right- and left-handed trabeculotomes (Harms or McPherson)	• 6–0 nylon suture
	• 9–0 polyglactin suture
	• 10–0 polyglactin suture
• Sharp triangular or paracentesis blade	• 10–0 polyglactin suture on tapered needle
• Angled Vannas scissors	• Prednisolone acetate 1% drops
• Fine forceps such as 0.12-mm toothed or jeweler's forceps	• Moxifloxacin eye drop or bacitracin/polymyxin ointment
• #57 Beaver blade	

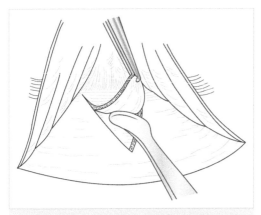

Fig. 16.1 A triangular limbus-based scleral flap is created.

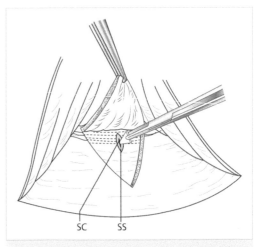

SC   SS

Fig. 16.2 A radial incision is made under the scleral flap from 1.0 mm anterior to 2.0 mm posterior to the limbal scleral junction. SC, Schlemm's canal; SS, scleral spur.

6. A radial partial thickness incision is made with a paracentesis blade, initially partial thickness and under the scleral flap, from 1.0 mm anterior to 2.0 mm posterior to the limbal scleral junction (▶ Fig. 16.2).

7. With continued dissection, the circumferential fibers of the scleral spur should become evident at the posterior third of the radial wound with less dense circumferential fibers found immediately over Schlemm's canal (▶ Fig. 16.3). The tissue making up the outer wall of Schlemm's canal often appears dark green-black.

8. Successively deeper layers of sclera through the radial incision are dissected, eventually entering Schlemm's canal through its outer wall.

9. Magnification should be increased at the surgeon's discretion for final dissection into Schlemm's canal.

10. Upon entry, blood or aqueous humor may appear.

11. A short length of 6–0 nylon suture may be held with fine forceps, such as jeweler's forceps, and passed to the right and then to the left circumferentially to test for the presence of Schlemm's canal.

12. Angled Vannas scissors are used to enlarge both sides of the entry into Schlemm's canal by placing one blade of the scissors in Schlemm's canal and cutting circumferentially to the right and then to the left of the radial incision.

13. A trabeculotome is then used to incise the trabecular meshwork (trabeculum) by placing the distal arm of the instrument into Schlemm's canal, and using the proximal arm as a guide for the placement of the distal arm

(▶ Fig. 16.4). No resistance should be encountered with this maneuver.

14. Once the distal arm is in the canal, it is rotated into the anterior chamber over the surface of the iris to expose approximately three-fourths of the arm's length in the anterior chamber; there should be no resistance to this rotation.

   a) If the trabeculotome is rotated in a plane angulated posteriorly, the iris may be encountered. If it is rotated in a plane angulated anteriorly, resistance may be felt due to engagement of tissue approximating Schwalbe's line.

15. Partial collapse of the anterior chamber may occur with the first rotation of the arm, requiring re-formation or deepening of the anterior chamber before the same maneuver is performed on the opposite side of the radial incision.

16. After the trabeculotome is used on both sides of the radial incision, the overlying triangular scleral flap is closed using 10–0 polyglactin suture to maintain the anterior chamber.

17. The conjunctival peritomy is then closed at the corners to the limbus with 9–0 polyglactin suture. The relaxing conjunctival incisions are closed with interrupted 10–0 polyglactin suture on a tapered needle.[1]

16.8 Tips and Pearls

Recurrent hemorrhage is unusual but requires anterior chamber washout if complicated by increased IOP.

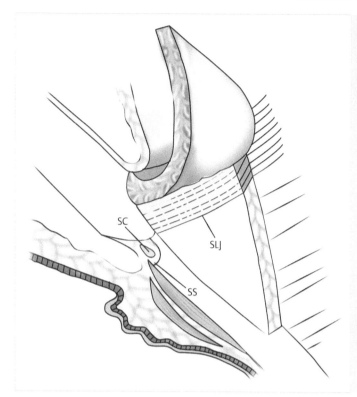

Fig. 16.3 With dissection, the circumferential fibers of the scleral spur become evident at the posterior third of the radial wound with less dense circumferential fibers found immediately over Schlemm's canal. SC, Schlemm's canal; SLJ, sclerolimbal junction; SS, scleral spur.

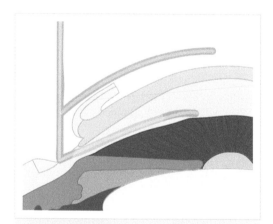

Fig. 16.4 The trabeculotome is used to incise the trabecular meshwork by placing the distal arm of the instrument into Schlemm's canal and using the proximal arm as a guide for the placement of the distal arm.

16.9 What to Avoid

- Injury to Descemet's membrane is possible if it is stripped as a result of anterior placement of the trabeculotome arm during rotation into the anterior chamber.
- Rotation of the trabculotome arm too far posteriorly can result in creation of iridodialysis or iridotomy.

16.10 Complications

- Hyphema
- Iridodialysis
- Iridotomy
- Stripping of Descemet's membrane

16.11 Postoperative Care

- A protective dressing with an eye pad and eye shield is placed after instillation of topical antibiotic and corticosteroid eye drops. The author uses prednisolone acetate 1% drops with moxifloxacin drops or polymyxin/bacitracin ointment. The dressing is kept in place for 24 hours, and postoperative drops are initiated on postoperative day 1. The eye shield should be continued through postoperative day 2.

- Head of bed elevation is important to allow the hyphema to settle inferiorly and prevent it from increasing in size by reducing episcleral venous pressure.

16.12 Acknowledgment

Special thanks to David S. Walton, MD for his guidance during the preparation of this chapter.

Reference

[1] Walton DS. Goniotomy, trabeculotomy, and goniosynechialysis. In: Higginbotham EJ, Lee DA, eds. Clinical Guide to Glaucoma Management. Woburn, MA: Butterworth-Heinemann; 2004:412–423

Section V

Procedures for Retinopathy of Prematurity

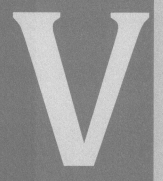

17 Laser Therapy for Retinopathy of Prematurity

Shilpa J. Desai and Michelle C. Liang

Summary

Retinopathy of prematurity (ROP) is a disease of very low birth weight premature infants involving abnormal vascularization and angiogenesis of the retina. With advancements in modern medicine, the survival of low birth weight infants is improving and, in turn, increasing the incidence of ROP. Without appropriate treatment, ROP can result in vision loss and blindness due to retinal detachment and temporal dragging of the retina.

Laser therapy (or laser photocoagulation) is a well-studied, safe, and effective treatment for Type I ROP. Understanding the indications, procedure, and potential side effects of this procedure allows for the successful treatment of ROP and avoidance of potentially sight-threatening complications.

Keywords: retinopathy of prematurity, Type I disease, Plus disease, laser therapy

17.1 Goals

- Induce regression of active retinopathy of prematurity (ROP).
- Avoid complications including macular dragging and tractional retinal detachment.

17.2 Advantages

Laser photocoagulation has numerous advantages over the alternative therapies for ROP: cryotherapy and anti-vascular endothelial growth factor (anti-VEGF) agents. Cryotherapy has largely been abandoned as a treatment for ROP as laser therapy has a higher success rate and improved visual outcomes compared to cryotherapy.[1] In addition, cryotherapy induces significantly greater amounts of myopia in the long term compared to laser.[2] Anti-VEGF therapy is a more recently developed treatment option for ROP but requires an intravitreal injection, carrying the additional risks of infection, bleeding, retinal detachment, and damage to the lens. The long-term systemic side effects of anti-VEGF agents in premature infants is also unknown.

17.3 Expectations

Successful laser therapy in patients with Type I ROP includes:

- Complete regression of active ROP
  - Without retinal detachment or distortion of posterior pole anatomy.

17.4 Key Principles

- Successful treatment of ROP requires an accurate and timely diagnosis of Type I ROP.
- Laser therapy (▶ Fig. 17.1 and ▶ Fig. 17.2) is indicated in premature infants with Type I ROP to prevent potential vision loss from untreated ROP.

17.5 Indications

There are two primary treatment guidelines for ROP. The multicenter Cryotherapy for Retinopathy of Prematurity (CRYO-ROP) study determined that treatment with cryotherapy should be initiated at threshold disease,[3] which was defined as at least 5 contiguous or 8 cumulative clock hours of stage 3 ROP in zone I or II with Plus disease.

Subsequently, the Early Treatment for Retinopathy of Prematurity (ETROP) study found better outcomes when treatment with laser therapy was initiated for Type I ROP, which was defined as[4,5]:

- Zone I, any stage ROP with Plus disease.
- Zone I, stage 3 ROP without Plus disease.
- Zone II, stage 2 or 3 ROP with Plus disease.

The ETROP study also defined Type II ROP as:
- Zone I, stage 1 or 2 ROP without Plus disease.
- Zone II, stage 3 ROP without Plus disease.

Type II ROP is recommended to be monitored weekly.

Neonates with stage 4 or 5 ROP (partial or total retinal detachment) require treatment with scleral buckle and vitrectomy. The outcomes for stages 4 and 5 ROP are guarded at best, and so appropriate initiation of therapy is key to preserving vision.

17.6 Contraindications

- Infants who are medically unstable for sedation and laser procedure.
- Poor view due to poor dilation or intraocular hemorrhage.

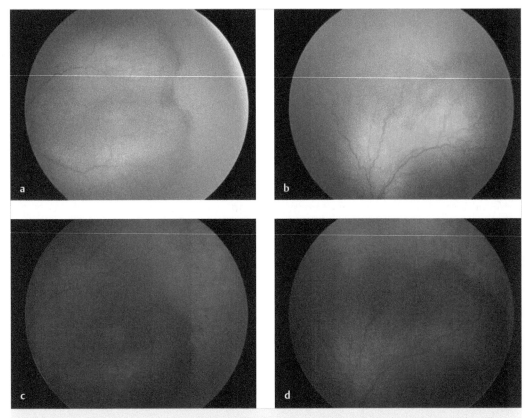

Fig. 17.1 **(a, b)** Patient with zone II, stage 3 retinopathy of prematurity (ROP) and Plus disease before and **(c, d)** immediately following laser.

17.7 Preoperative Preparation

ROP screening is performed based on the patient's gestational age at birth, birth weight, and clinical status with follow-up examinations and determination for treatment based on examination findings.[6] Screening examinations require dilation with cyclopentolate 0.2% and phenylephrine 1%, which are usually available as a combination drop. ROP is graded based on the location and severity of disease.

The location of retinal vascularization defines the zone:

- Zone I: A circle twice the distance from the center of the disc to the center of the macula and centered on the optic disc.
- Zone II: The area encircling zone I, extending to the nasal ora.
- Zone III: The remaining crescent of temporal retina.

The stage of disease is determined by the appearance of the region between the vascular and avascular retina:

- Stage 1: Flat demarcation line.
- Stage 2: Elevated ridge.
- Stage 3: Ridge with extraretinal neovascularization.
- Stage 4: Partial retinal detachment.
- Stage 5: Total retinal detachment.

Plus disease is defined as the presence of dilated and tortuous vessels in two or more quadrants, and is often a deciding factor for treatment. Pre-plus disease may be noted as well, which is arteriolar tortuosity and venular dilation that is greater than normal but does not meet the definition of Plus disease. Aggressive posterior ROP (AP-ROP) involves tortuous vessels in all quadrants out of proportion to the extent of peripheral retinopathy, progresses rapidly, and has a poorer prognosis.

Once a neonate has any stage of ROP, the findings should be discussed with the patient's family. This prepares the family for the potential need for future treatment. If laser therapy is indicated, then

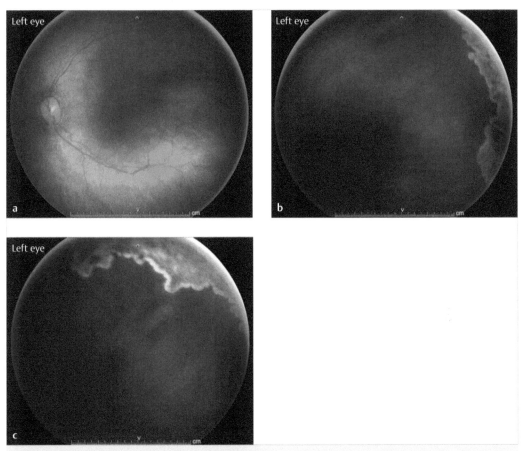

Fig. 17.2 The same patient 1 month after retinopathy of prematurity (ROP) laser showing **(a)** regression of Plus disease and **(b, c)** peripheral stage 3 ROP.

treatment recommendations, risks of treatment, and potential prognosis should be discussed.

17.8 Operative Technique

Laser treatment for ROP can be performed in the operating room under general anesthesia (▶ Fig. 17.3) or at the bedside with monitored sedation. The optimal location depends on the stability of the infant and the preferences of the physician administering the anesthesia and the treating ophthalmologist. Coordination of care with the treatment team is crucial to ensure the best possible outcome for the patient.

1. The baby should be positioned for the surgeon to be able to complete the laser treatment as efficiently as possible. The surgeon should have the ability to move around the infant circumferentially to allow for lasering of the entire retinal periphery.[7]

2. An indirect diode laser with 810 nm wavelength is recommended, as the diode laser has a decreased incidence of cataract formation at 0.003% compared to argon laser at 1 to 6%.[8,9,10] A 28-diopter condensing lens is the best lens to use for the larger field of view. A neonatal eyelid speculum and scleral depressor are also used.

3. The laser is applied transpupillary in a near confluent pattern throughout the avascular retina to the ora serrata for 360 degrees. The laser burn should be dull-white in color. Typical settings are between 150 and 250 mW, pulse duration of 100 to 200 ms, with only 0.5–1 burn width between each laser spot. In cases of aggressive or persistent ROP, laser can also be applied posterior to the ridge.[11] Generally, 2,000 to 3,000 spots are applied for the

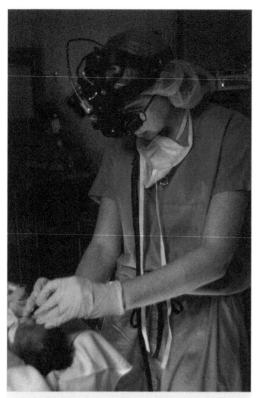

Fig. 17.3 Application of laser photocoagulation to a premature baby in the operating room setting.

treatment of zone II disease, with additional spots for zone I disease.

4. It is easiest to begin the laser at the most accessible and concerning area first, which is usually the temporal ridge. The laser can then be continued from the ridge anteriorly with gentle depression on the globe and continued for 360 degrees.

5. Before concluding the laser treatment, the periphery should be re-examined for any skip areas, using a scleral depressor to ensure that treatment extends to the ora serrata for 360 degrees.

17.9 Tips and Pearls

- The steepness and small size of the cornea require a more vertical viewing angle than in adults. Avoid a horizontal viewing angle.
- Laser treatment in infants is more challenging than in adults and can take 60 to 90 minutes.

17.10 What to Avoid

- Avoid depressing the globe too posteriorly as this will make viewing the ora more difficult. The ora serrata is only 1.0 mm beyond the limbus in infants compared to 3.5 to 4 mm beyond the limbus in adults.
- Avoid depressing the globe excessively or releasing pressure on the globe suddenly, as these maneuvers can cause pupillary constriction and vitreous hemorrhage.
- Avoid desiccation of the cornea by lubricating the cornea throughout treatment with saline solution.

17.11 Complications

- The most common complication of ROP laser is continued progression of disease, which may present as lack of regression of the ROP ridge, persistence of Plus disease, neovascularization of the iris, or vitreous hemorrhage. In this situation, examine the patient carefully for skip areas which may be continuing to produce VEGF. Fluorescein angiography can be useful to evaluate for untreated areas of avascular retina.
- Inflammation may occur as a result of both the ROP disease and the laser treatment. If an exudative retinal detachment develops, it can be treated with subconjunctival dexamethasone (2.5 mg per eye) or systemic corticosteroids to quell the inflammatory response.[12] The dose of systemic corticosteroids should be discussed with the primary team; case reports suggest a dose of 0.6 mg/kg/day.[13]
- Lens opacities can occur with either argon or diode laser;[14,15] however, the rate is lower with the diode laser.
- Development of hyphema has also been reported.[16]
- Aggressive laser using excessive total energy can also lead to anterior segment complications including hypotony, iris atrophy,[17] and phthisis.[18,19] Patients treated at a younger postmenstrual age may have an increased risk of anterior segment complications.[20]

17.12 Postoperative Care

- Continue cyclopentolate 0.2% and phenylephrine 1%, usually available as a combination drop, three times daily to prevent synechiae formation from intraocular inflammation. Prednisolone acetate 1% four times daily, as well as a topical antibiotic for infectious prophylaxis, can also be added. Topical therapy is started immediately following laser treatment and continued for 5 to 7 days.

- Re-examine the patient 24 to 48 hours after laser treatment and then monitor weekly until the ROP regresses. In addition to regression of the neovascular ridge, other signs of regression include improved pupillary dilation, resolution of iris neovascularization, clearing of retinal or vit-reous hemorrhage, and regression of Plus disease.
- In persistent disease, additional laser posterior to the ridge or anti-VEGF therapy can be considered.
- Once the ROP is regressed and stable, the patient should be monitored at least yearly.
- In the long term, visual field loss and increased rates of strabismus and high myopia are also seen. All patients with a history of prematurity and ROP should also be evaluated by a pediatric ophthalmologist.

References

[1] Paysse EA, Lindsey JL, Coats DK, Contant CF, Jr, Steinkuller PG. Therapeutic outcomes of cryotherapy versus transpupillary diode laser photocoagulation for threshold retinopathy of prematurity. J AAPOS. 1999; 3(4):234–240

[2] Connolly BP, Ng EY, McNamara JA, Regillo CD, Vander JF, Tasman W. A comparison of laser photocoagulation with cryotherapy for threshold retinopathy of prematurity at 10 years: part 2. Refractive outcome. Ophthalmology. 2002; 109 (5):936–941

[3] Cryotherapy for Retinopathy of Prematurity Cooperative Group. Multicenter trial of cryotherapy for retinopathy of prematurity: ophthalmological outcomes at 10 years. Arch Ophthalmol. 2001; 119(8):1110–1118

[4] Early Treatment for Retinopathy of Prematurity Cooperative Group. Revised indications for the treatment of retinopathy of prematurity: results of the early treatment for retinopathy of prematurity randomized trial. Arch Ophthalmol. 2003; 121(12):1684–1694

[5] Good WV, Early Treatment for Retinopathy of Prematurity Cooperative Group. Final results of the Early Treatment for Retinopathy of Prematurity (ETROP) randomized trial. Trans Am Ophthalmol Soc. 2004; 102:233–248, discussion 248–250

[6] Kothari NA, Berrocal AM. Retinopathy of prematurity. In: Duker JS, Liang MC, eds. Anti-VEGF Use in Ophthalmology. Thorofare, NJ: SLACK Inc; 2017:143–150

[7] Kychenthal BA, Dorta SP, eds. Retinopathy of Prematurity: Current Diagnosis and Management. Cham, Switzerland: Springer; 2017

[8] Paysse EA, Miller A, Brady McCreery KM, Coats DK. Acquired cataracts after diode laser photocoagulation for threshold retinopathy of prematurity. Ophthalmology. 2002; 109(9): 1662–1665

[9] O'Neil JW, Hutchinson AK, Saunders RA, Wilson ME. Acquired cataracts after argon laser photocoagulation for retinopathy of prematurity. J AAPOS. 1998; 2(1):48–51

[10] Christiansen SP, Bradford JD. Cataract following diode laser photoablation for retinopathy of prematurity. Arch Ophthalmol 1997;115(2):275–276

[11] Ells AL, Gole GA, Lloyd Hildebrand P, Ingram A, Wilson CM, Geoff Williams R. Posterior to the ridge laser treatment for severe stage 3 retinopathy of prematurity. Eye (Lond). 2013; 27(4):525–530

[12] Moinuddin O, Bonaffini S, Besirli CG. Exudative retinal detachment following laser photocoagulation for retinopathy of prematurity: a rare complication. Ophthalmic Surg Lasers Imaging Retina. 2019; 50(4):242–246

[13] Moshfeghi DM, Silva RA, Berrocal AM. Exudative retinal detachment following photocoagulation in older premature infants for retinopathy of prematurity: description and management. Retina. 2014; 34(1):83–86

[14] Drack AV, Burke JP, Pulido JS, Keech RV. Transient punctate lenticular opacities as a complication of argon laser photoablation in an infant with retinopathy of prematurity. Am J Ophthalmol. 1992; 113(5):583–584

[15] Capone A, Jr, Drack AV. Transient lens changes after diode laser retinal photoablation for retinopathy of prematurity. Am J Ophthalmol. 1994; 118(4):533–535

[16] Simons BD, Wilson MC, Hertle RW, Schaefer DB. Bilateral hyphemas and cataracts after diode laser retinal photoabla-tion for retinopathy of prematurity. J Pediatr Ophthalmol Strabismus. 1998; 35(3):185–187

[17] Kaiser RS, Trese MT. Iris atrophy, cataracts, and hypotony following peripheral ablation for threshold retinopathy of prematurity. Arch Ophthalmol. 2001; 119(4):615–617

[18] Lambert SR, Capone A, Jr, Cingle KA, Drack AV. Cataract and phthisis bulbi after laser photoablation for threshold retinopathy of prematurity. Am J Ophthalmol. 2000; 129(5): 585–591

[19] Ibarra MS, Capone A, Jr. Retinopathy of prematurity and ante-rior segment complications. Ophthalmol Clin North Am. 2004; 17(4):577–582, vii

[20] Salgado CM, Celik Y, VanderVeen DK. Anterior segment com-plications after diode laser photocoagulation for prethreshold retinopathy of prematurity. Am J Ophthalmol. 2010; 150(1): 6–9.e2

18 Anti-Vascular Endothelial Growth Factor Therapy for Retinopathy of Prematurity

Michelle C. Liang and Shilpa J. Desai

Summary

Retinopathy of prematurity (ROP), associated with low gestational age and birth weight, is a leading cause of childhood blindness worldwide. Treatment of Type I ROP results in improved visual acuity outcomes and decreased rates of retinal detachment. Laser photocoagulation to the avascular retina has largely replaced cryotherapy as the mainstay of treatment, but the use of anti-vascular endothelial growth factor (anti-VEGF) agents has increased as an alternative to laser therapy within the last decade.

At this time, no anti-VEGF medications are FDA-approved for the treatment of ROP, so all such treatments are performed off-label. There is a large variability in practice patterns, and additional studies are needed to determine the optimal approach to treating ROP with anti-VEGF agents. There are no definitive guidelines for when anti-VEGF treatment is indicated or when and for how long to monitor patients after treatment. There is also no consensus on the definition of ROP recurrence, whether this includes worsening of Plus disease or recurrence of stage 3 disease, and when and how to treat recurrence. Finally, although available studies suggest no adverse effects on medical or neurodevelopmental outcomes with the use of anti-VEGF therapy, long-term follow-up is not yet available.

With the limitations mentioned above, this section discusses the use of anti-VEGF medications in the treatment of ROP and detailed techniques of intravitreal injections in a neonate, with attention to how they differ from intravitreal injections in adults.

Keywords: retinopathy of prematurity, Type I disease, Plus disease, anti-vascular endothelial growth factor therapy, intravitreal injection

18.1 Goals

- Induce regression of active retinopathy of prematurity (ROP).
- Avoid complications including macular dragging and tractional retinal detachment.

18.2 Advantages

The treatment options for Type I ROP include laser photocoagulation, which has largely replaced cryotherapy, and anti-VEGF therapy. Although it has been the standard of care for many years, laser photocoagulation has its drawbacks. Very posterior disease requires retinal ablation near the fovea and macula, and infants with aggressive posterior ROP (AP-ROP) can rapidly progress despite laser treatment. Laser photocoagulation also has known complications including visual field loss and increased rates of strabismus and high myopia.

Anti-VEGF agents have more recently been used to treat ROP without the destruction of retinal tissue. Specifically, it can be used to treat posterior disease to avoid laser treatment near the macula, and it may induce regression of AP-ROP more quickly than laser photocoagulation. In addition, it has been used as an adjunctive treatment in ROP that progresses despite laser therapy. Numerous case reports and case series on using anti-VEGF agents for ROP have been published, and the Bevacizumab Eliminates the Angiogenic Threat of Retinopathy of Prematurity (BEAT-ROP) and RAnibizumab Compared with Laser Therapy for the Treatment of INfants BOrn Prematurely With Retinopathy of Prematurity (RAINBOW) randomized controlled trials showed the benefit of bevacizumab and ranibizumab, respectively, for the treatment of ROP.[1]

BEAT-ROP was the first prospective, randomized, multicenter trial that compared monotherapy with intravitreal bevacizumab to conventional diode laser for infants with stage 3 ROP with Plus disease in zone I or posterior zone II. Eyes treated with 0.625 mg intravitreal bevacizumab had lower rates of recurrence, although this was significant only in eyes with zone I disease (6% vs. 42% at 54 weeks), not those with zone II disease. It was also noted that recurrence after treatment with bevacizumab typically occurred later than after laser treatment (mean 16 weeks vs. 6.2 weeks), with recurrence after the 54-week follow-up visit not uncommon.[2]

The RAINBOW trial compared intravitreal ranibizumab to laser therapy for the treatment of ROP. Primary outcome measures included the absence of active ROP and unfavorable structural outcome at 24 weeks. Data from this study showed that 80% of patients who received 0.2 mg ranibizumab met criteria for success, compared to 66% who received laser. Ranibizumab led to higher success rates for ROP in both zone I and zone II disease.[3]

Although both laser photocoagulation and intravitreal injection require well-trained ophthalmologists, treatment with intravitreal anti-VEGF medication is arguably easier and relies less on the skill of the ophthalmologist once the medication is in the eye. It can be administered quickly at the bedside with local anesthesia, using less equipment compared too laser therapy. In addition, neonates most at risk for ROP requiring treatment may be too unstable to undergo a longer procedure with sedation, which is typically required for laser treatment. Intravitreal injections can also be administered in patients with small pupils or a dense vitreous hemorrhage, which may render laser treatment difficult or impossible to perform. Additionally, by avoiding laser treatment, the area of viable retinal tissue may be increased, reducing the incidence of peripheral visual field loss and laser-associated myopia.

18.3 Expectations

Successful anti-VEGF therapy in patients with Type I ROP includes:
- Complete regression of active ROP:
  - Without retinal detachment or distortion of posterior pole anatomy.
- Continued growth of retinal vasculature anteriorly into zone II in more posterior disease and toward the retinal periphery.

Expectations of anti-VEGF therapy should be discussed in detail with the patient's family. Although there has been success in the treatment of ROP with anti-VEGF agents, infants must be monitored weekly for disease recurrence and additional treatment that may be needed. Incomplete retinal vascularization and late recurrence are not uncommon, and compliance with follow-up may be a factor when considering which treatment option best suits the patient and also the patient's family.

18.4 Key Principles

There is currently no universal protocol for intravitreal injection in the prematurely born neonatal population, and there are no definitive recommendations on sclerotomy placement due to uncertainty and variation of the location of the ora serrata in these patients.

There is a high risk of touching the lens with intravitreal injection in an infant compared to adult patients, as well as a risk of inadvertent traction on the vitreous base.

18.5 Indications

The treatment of ROP with anti-VEGF therapy is not standardized and can vary between treating ophthalmologists.

Infants who may benefit the most from anti-VEGF therapy include those with:
- Posterior disease (zone I or posterior zone II) (▶ Fig. 18.1).
- AP-ROP (▶ Fig. 18.2).
- Persistent active ROP despite laser therapy (▶ Fig. 18.3).

As well as infants:
- Who may be too unstable to undergo laser therapy with sedation.
- With an inadequate view for laser therapy.

18.6 Contraindications

Although there do not appear to be absolute contraindications to intravitreal anti-VEGF injection, pre-existing ocular conditions may warrant special consideration[4]:
- Active external infection, including conjunctivitis, hordeolum, or cellulitis.
- Elevated intraocular pressure or glaucoma.
- Active uveitis.

These conditions are less commonly seen in the neonatal population compared to adults, and treatment of Type I ROP typically must be administered in a timely manner to reduce the risk of worsening and progression to retinal detachment or other possibly vision-threatening structural abnormalities.

18.7 Preoperative Preparation

Preoperative preparation is similar to that of an intravitreal injection in an adult (▶ Fig. 18.4). Betadine 5% is used prior to the injection to reduce the incidence of infection.[4] A sterile eyelid speculum and sterile calipers are used, and a scleral depressor or toothed forceps may be helpful to fixate the globe.

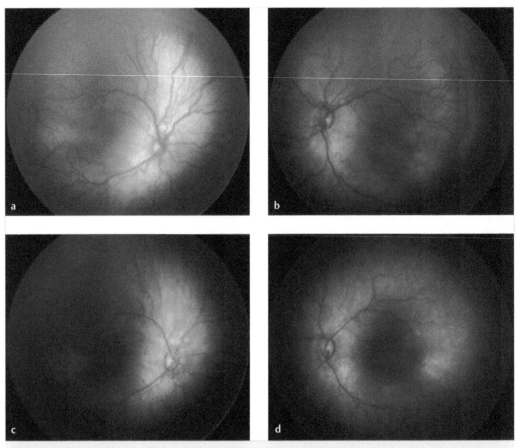

Fig. 18.1 Reduced Plus disease and increased retinal vascularization after intravitreal ranibizumab monotherapy. **(a, b)** Fundus photographs prior to treatment demonstrate Plus disease, stage 3 retinopathy of prematurity (ROP) in posterior zone II, and avascular peripheral retina. **(c, d)** Fundus photography 3 weeks after treatment shows regression of the Plus disease and peripheral ROP as well as increased retinal vascularization into the periphery.

18.8 Operative Technique

Intravitreal injection of anti-VEGF medication can be performed at the bedside or in an operating room under local anesthesia. There is large variability in practice patterns regarding the sterile technique for intravitreal injections, even in adults, especially in regards to the use of an eyelid speculum, gloves, and/or masks.[4] It is recommended that injections in newborns be performed under aseptic conditions.

The choice of local anesthesia is according to surgeon's preference but includes topical proparacaine, lidocaine or tetracaine gel, and subconjunctival lidocaine. Many surgeons recommend pre-injection topical anesthetic eye drops or gel, and some recommend avoidance of subconjunctival lidocaine which may distort the ocular anatomy.

1. The eye is prepped with 5% betadine.
2. An eyelid speculum is recommended to keep the eyelids and eyelashes away from the injection site. A caliper is used to mark 1.0 mm posterior to the limbus in the inferior or inferotemporal quadrant, depending on exposure and surgeon's preference (▶ Fig. 18.5). The selected anti-VEGF agent is injected using a small-gauge needle (30 gauge or smaller) on a 1-mL syringe, with careful attention to not place the needle too far into the vitreous cavity and to aim posteriorly without damaging the lens or the retina.
3. Sterile saline can be used following the procedure to irrigate the eye and avoid betadine toxicity to the ocular surface.

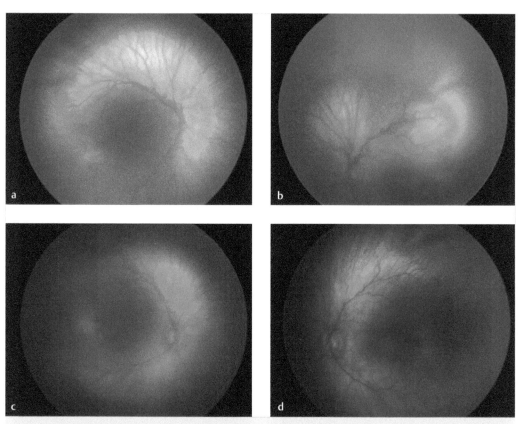

Fig. 18.2 Advanced posterior retinopathy of prematurity (ROP) before and after intravitreal ranibizumab. **(a, b)** Fundus photograph shows tortuous vessels and flat stage 3 disease within zone I. **(c, d)** Fundus photograph 2 weeks after intravitreal ranibizumab demonstrates resolution of tortuous vasculature and stage 3 disease.

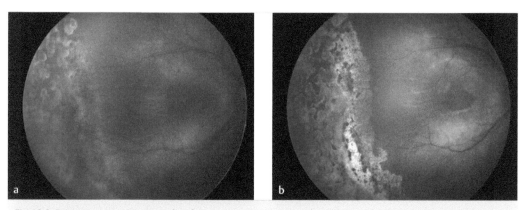

Fig. 18.3 Persistent stage 3 retinopathy of prematurity (ROP) despite laser therapy. **(a)** Fundus photograph reveals persistent stage 3 disease temporally despite confluent surrounding laser therapy. **(b)** There is resolution of the stage 3 disease 1 week after intravitreal ranibizumab.

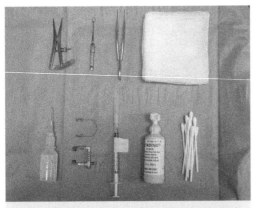

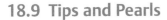

Fig. 18.4 Suggested instrument tray for bedside intravitreal injection which includes povidone-iodine 5%, sterile eyelid speculum, sterile calipers, anti-vascular endothelial growth factor (anti-VEGF) in a 1 mL syringe with a 30-gauge needle, sterile cotton-tipped applicators, balanced salt solution, and gauze. A scleral depressor or 0.12-mm forceps may also be used to help with globe fixation.

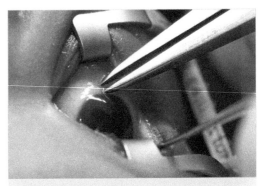

Fig. 18.5 Preparing for intravitreal injection. An eyelid speculum is used to keep the eyelashes away from the injection site. Sterile calipers are used to mark 1.0 mm posterior to the inferior limbus.

18.9 Tips and Pearls

- Optimal dosing and needle size have not yet been defined. BEAT-ROP used a 31-gauge, approximately 8-mm needle with half the adult dose of bevacizumab (0.625 mg). The RAINBOW trial used a 30-gauge, approximately 12-mm needle with 0.1 and 0.2 mg doses of ranibizumab. Alternatively, a 32-gauge, 4-mm needle may decrease the risk of iatrogenic retinal breaks and lenticular injury.[5]
- A small volume syringe for the anti-VEGF medication is ideal for control of the injection and to avoid incorrect volume delivery.
- Injection sites can range from 0.5 to 2 mm posterior to the limbus, with a maximum of 2.5 mm, as utilized in BEAT-ROP.
- Aim the needle away from the lens and straight into the vitreous to avoid full-thickness retinal injury.

18.10 What to Avoid

Prematurely born newborns have an underdeveloped pars plana and short anteroposterior globe diameter. This may predispose them to iatrogenic anterior retinal breaks after intravitreal injection. Standard 0.5-inch (12.7 mm) needles may result in inadvertent retinal injury, and the large size of the lens relative to the globe size poses a greater risk of lens injury if the angle of entry is not pointed toward the optic nerve. These risks may be even greater because injections are done with local anesthesia, and newborns may move during the injection. Infection may also occur at a higher rate due to underdeveloped immunity and the presence of systemic comorbidities often seen in patients with severe ROP.[6]

18.11 Complications

Ocular:
- Cataract or other injury to the lens.
- Subconjunctival or intraocular hemorrhage.
- Retinal tear or detachment.
- Elevated intraocular pressure.
- Endophthalmitis.
- Incomplete retinal vascular development:
  - Further studies are needed to evaluate when and how vascularization occurs following anti-VEGF therapy.
  - Fluorescein angiography can improve the sensitivity of diagnosis of ROP, as it may allow better assessment of peripheral avascular zones and the need for additional therapy.
- Persistent or recurrent ROP (▶ Fig. 18.6 and ▶ Fig. 18.7):
  - Laser therapy or additional anti-VEGF therapy may be required in patients who do not respond to initial anti-VEGF therapy or for those in whom disease recurs or worsens.
- Progressive tractional retinal detachment[6]

Although treatment with anti-VEGF agents appears to be safe, efficacious, and well-tolerated in premature infants with ROP, further research is needed to determine the optimal treatment regimen and potential long-term systemic side effects.

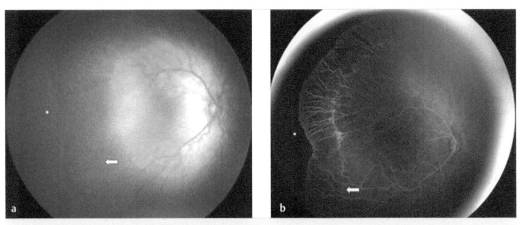

Fig. 18.6 Recurrent retinopathy of prematurity (ROP) after intravitreal ranibizumab. **(a)** Fundus photograph demonstrates recurrence of stage 2 disease in the temporal periphery (*asterisks*). The edge of the vascularized retina has progressed, but **(b)** there is leakage at the previous demarcation line (*arrows*).

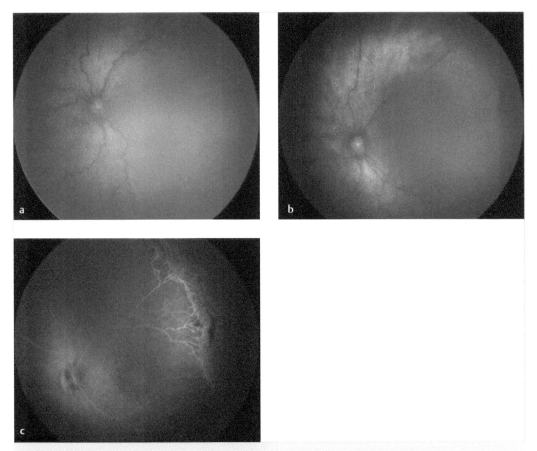

Fig. 18.7 Persistent retinopathy of prematurity (ROP) after intravitreal ranibizumab. **(a)** Fundus photograph reveals tortuous vessels, stage 3 ROP in posterior zone II, and avascular peripheral retina. **(b, c)** There is persistent, active disease 1 week after treatment for which laser treatment was performed.

18.12 Postoperative Care

Following intravitreal injection, topical antibiotic (four times a day), corticosteroid (four times a day), and cycloplegic eye drops (two times a day) are usually recommended for 1 week. Additional care must be taken to keep the eyes clean and avoid contamination of the eye after the procedure.

References

[1] Kothari NA, Berrocal AM. Retinopathy of prematurity. In: Duker JS, Liang MC, eds. Anti-VEGF Use in Ophthalmology. Thorofare, NJ: SLACK Inc; 2017:143–150

[2] Mintz-Hittner HA, Kennedy KA, Chuang AZ, BEAT-ROP Cooperative Group. Efficacy of intravitreal bevacizumab for stage 3 + retinopathy of prematurity. N Engl J Med. 2011; 364(7): 603–615

[3] Stahl A, Lepore D, Fielder A, et al. Ranibizumab versus laser therapy for the treatment of very low birthweight infants with retinopathy of prematurity (RAINBOW): an open-label randomised controlled trial. Lancet. 2019; 394(10208): 1551–1559

[4] Muakkassa N, Klein K, Reichel E. Intravitreal delivery. In: Duker JS, Liang MC, eds. Anti-VEGF Use in Ophthalmology. Thorofare, NJ: SLACK Inc; 2017:47–56

[5] Wright LM, Vrcek IM, Scribbick FW, III, Chang EY, Harper CA, III. Technique for infant intravitreal injection in treatment of retinopathy of prematurity. Retina. 2017; 37(11): 2188–2190

[6] Yonekawa Y, Wu WC, Nitulescu CE, et al. Progressive retinal detachment in infants with retinopathy of prematurity treated with intravitreal bevacizumab or ranibizumab. Retina. 2018; 38(6):1079–1083

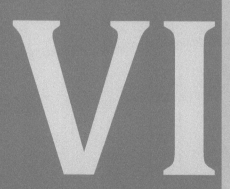

Section VI

Examination Under Anesthesia

VI

19 Preparations for Examinations under Anesthesia

Sylvia H. Yoo

Summary

Examinations under anesthesia are required when a child cannot be adequately examined in the eye clinic for potentially vision-threatening eye disease. Additional testing may also be indicated while the patient is sedated.

Keywords: examination under anesthesia, intraocular pressure, ocular biometry, electroretinogram

19.1 Goals

Obtaining as complete an examination as possible while the patient is sedated.

19.2 Advantages

An examination under anesthesia can provide the information needed for appropriate treatment planning in a patient who is otherwise unable to be adequately examined in the clinic.

19.3 Expectations

Adequate anesthesia to complete the eye examination and any additional planned testing. Strabismus cannot be accurately evaluated while the patient is under anesthesia, but forced duction testing may be performed.

19.4 Key Principles and Preoperative Preparation

Determine the elements of the examination and testing needed during the examination under anesthesia when planning and scheduling the case. If possible and if needed for the patient's examination, instill dilating eye drops preoperatively to decrease the time under anesthesia.

19.5 Indications

Potentially vision-threatening eye disease that cannot be adequately evaluated in the office due to lack of cooperation, or which requires testing that will not be tolerated by the patient while awake.

19.6 Contraindications

Some patients whose examinations are limited in the office may have underlying systemic disease that put them at greater anesthesia risk. The indications for the examination under anesthesia should be discussed with the patient's family, pediatrician, as well as the anesthesia team.

19.7 Operative Technique

In coordination with the anesthesiologist, measure the intraocular pressure with a Tono-Pen or a Perkins tonometer as soon as it is safe for the patient during induction of anesthesia. Following induction of anesthesia, usually after the airway is secured, the Perkins tonometer can be used to measure the intraocular pressure if it was not used for the initial measurement, keeping in mind that the anesthetic agents that were used may affect the measurements.

The following measurements and examination elements are subsequently performed using the appropriate instruments, as indicated:
1. Central corneal thickness with a pachymeter.
2. Corneal diameters, both horizontal and vertical, with calipers.
3. Slit lamp examination with a portable slit lamp.
4. Gonioscopy can be performed with a portable slit lamp or a surgical microscope.
5. Dilated fundoscopic examination of the posterior pole and periphery using a scleral depressor or cotton-tip applicator to rotate the eye.
6. Cycloplegic retinoscopy using a retinoscope and retinoscopy bars or loose lenses.

Additional testing may include:
1. Ocular biometry
   - Keratometry with a handheld keratometer.
   - Axial length measurements with immersion. A-scan ultrasound, performed after keratometry.
2. Electroretinogram.
3. Fundus photography.
4. Fluorescein angiography.
5. Portable optical coherence tomography.

19.8 Tips and Pearls

- During cycloplegic retinoscopy, the eye alignment should grossly be in primary gaze, and the working distance should be approximately the same as that used in the office; a stepstool can be helpful to maintain the usual working distance. Otherwise, the final refraction is adjusted as judged by the examiner.
- Prepare an examination sheet to be able to quickly record the measurements in an organized manner. The timing of the intraocular pressure measurement, in relation to induction of anesthesia, should be noted.

19.9 What to Avoid

Plan ahead to ensure that all equipment and staff for specialized testing are available to avoid prolonging anesthesia.

19.10 Complications

Electroretinogram testing may be affected by the anesthetic agents used[1] and by the operating room setting, namely, the inability to completely darken the room for scotopic responses. This may result in an electroretinogram that is difficult to interpret, but significantly abnormal waveforms can be identified and are helpful in the diagnostic workup of patients with suspected retinal dystrophies. If fluorescein angiography is performed, there is a low risk of allergy to the fluorescein dye. Otherwise, the primary risk of an examination under anesthesia is the risk of undergoing general anesthesia.

19.11 Postoperative Care

Discussion of examination findings and planning for treatments and follow-up examinations with the patient's family is done following the examination under anesthesia. The possible need for future examinations under anesthesia is also discussed, if applicable.

Reference

[1] Tremblay F, Parkinson JE, Lalonde MR. Anesthesia and electroretinography. IOVS. 2003; 44:1897

Index

Note: Page numbers set **bold** or *italic* indicate headings or figures, respectively.